THE HEALTHY
Renegade
PASTOR

ABANDONING AVERAGE IN YOUR HEALTH AND WELLNESS

NELSON SEARCY
STEVE REYNOLDS & JENNIFER DYKES HENSON

Library of Congress Cataloging-in-Publication Data
Searcy, Nelson
The Healthy Renegade Pastor : abandoning average in your health and wellness /
Nelson Searcy; with Steve Reynolds and Jennifer Dykes Henson
p. cm.
Includes bibliographical references.
ISBN 978-0-9885241-1-8
1. Religion – Christian Ministry – Pastoral Resources

The website addresses recommended throughout this book are offered as a resource to you.

Unless otherwise noted, all Scripture quotations are taken from the *Holy Bible*, New Living Translation, copyright © 1996, 2007 by Tyndale House Foundation. Used by permission of Tyndale House Publishers, Inc., Carol Stream, Illinois 60188. All rights reserved; MSG are taken from *The Message*, copyright © 1993, 2002 by Eugene H. Peterson. Used by permission of NavPress Publishing Group; NIV are taken from the Holy Bible, New International Version˙ NIV˙, copyright © 1973, 2011 by Biblica, Inc. ™ Used by permission of Zondervan. All rights reserved worldwide; NKJV are taken from the New King James Version®, copyright © 1982 by Thomas Nelson, Inc. Used by permission. All rights reserved.

The author has added italics to Scripture quotations for emphasis.

Printed in the United States of America
First Edition 2015

To all of the pastors who are ready to get healthier, live more fully,
and accomplish the unique purposes God has set before them.

Authors' Note: Through the process of writing of this book, the three of us have taken our own health to a new level. As we've collaborated with one another and shared our stories of abandoning average in our physical health, we have learned much from each other's personal journeys. While the thoughts, anecdotes and principles presented in these pages represent the contributions of all three authors, we've chosen to fuse those contributions into one voice for clarity's sake. **Unless otherwise noted, the voice in the pages ahead is Nelson's.**

Contents

SPREADING THE WELLNESS

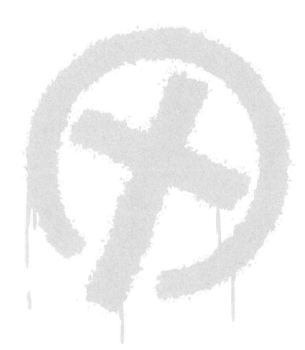

Abandoning Average

1

Abandoning Average:
A Tale of Two Pastors

If you want to be successful in life and you have no role models, look at what the majority of people are doing and do the opposite. The majority is always wrong.

EARL NIGHTINGALE

Do not be deceived: God cannot be mocked. A man reaps what he sows.

GALATIANS 6:7

Tired. Stressed. Sick. Overweight. Do these words describe you? For the vast majority of pastors, they are the norm. Over the course of our years as church leaders, too many of us have sacrificed our health and wellbeing on the altar of ministry. We have lost the vibrancy—and the waistlines—we once had, opting instead for the poor, counterfeit version of health that has become acceptable in our culture. It's no secret that, as a nation, we are facing a health crisis. I'm sure you've heard the statistics, but let me remind you of just a couple:

- Time trend forecasts predict that by 2030, 51% of the population will be obese.[1]

- Researchers predict that such rates of obesity will result in an additional $66 billion in health care expenditures, 7.8 million new cases of diabetes, 6.8 million new cases of stroke and heart disease, and 539,000 new cancer diagnoses.[2]

Those are staggering numbers, but they are just the tip of the iceberg for you and me. Among church leaders, the picture is even bleaker:

- A recent Pulpit and Pew study of 2500 clergy found that 76% were overweight or obese.[3]

- Clergy have one of the highest death rates from heart disease of any occupation.[4]

- 40% of pastors say they are depressed at times, and worn out "some or most of the time."[5]

We tell ourselves all kinds of lies to justify how far we've fallen:

- *I'm not that overweight. Lots of people are much bigger than me.*

- *I don't have time to work out.*

- *I'm busy doing God's work, so he'll take care of my body.*

- *When it's my time to go, I'll die. There's not much I can do about it in the meantime.*

- *This condition runs in my family. It doesn't have anything to do with my lifestyle.*

- *All pastors are stressed out. It's part of the job.*

At first, we believe ourselves. We convince ourselves that we are doing okay compared to the next guy and we forge ahead, blinders firmly in place. But eventually, the consequences of years of poor health decisions catch up. It's inevitable. When they do, our bodies suffer and our ministries suffer. We end up fat, chronically sick, dependent on pills to regulate our bodies' systems, and stressed to the point of burn-out or even depression. None of this is good for us, our churches, or God's greater kingdom. No matter how much we like to try, we can't get away from the truth Paul spelled out so clearly in Galatians:

> *Do not be deceived: God cannot be mocked.*
> ***A man reaps what he sows.***
> —Galatians 6:7 (emphasis added)

Two Paths Diverged

The lives of two great pastors I know provide the perfect case study for the slippery slope to ill health that can happen so easily in ministry. If you read *The Renegade Pastor: Abandoning Average in Your Life and Ministry*, then you've met these two before. In case you haven't, allow me to reintroduce them:

Alex and Rob are both faithful, well-intentioned guys whose lives were on similar trajectories when they were young. They were both called to ministry during college and went on to attend comparable seminaries. Now, each of them pastors a mid-sized church in the Midwest. Like you and me, both Alex and Rob started out in ministry with grand visions of what the future would bring. Each was in his prime, healthy and vibrant. They both wanted to change lives and grow the kingdom. Over the years, though, Alex and Rob's paths have diverged—both in terms of the churches and personal lives they have led and in their ability to fulfill their calling due to their different health journeys. (To learn more about how Alex and Rob's ministries and personal lives have taken drastically different paths, read *The Renegade Pastor: Abandoning Average in Your Life and Ministry*, Regal, 2013.)

Alex and Rob both still want to be on fire for God's work and to be filled with the energy and vitality it takes to do that work well, but Alex is beginning to face some health challenges that are slowing him down. With each passing year, he finds himself thicker around the middle, less energetic and less able to get excited about running after what God has called him to. On the other hand, Rob wakes up every morning feeling strong and refreshed, ready to use the full measure of his life to passionately pursue the visions God has given him. What's the difference?

Maybe the pseudo-last names I've given them for purposes of this case study will be a clue: Alex Average allows the busyness of his days to direct the decisions he makes (or fails to make) about his health. Because he's so consumed with the pressures of ministry and home life, his physical wellbeing is on autopilot. He eats whatever he can grab between meetings; he never has time to get to the gym; and he's constantly stressed as he scrambles to get his message together for the upcoming weekend. (Go to HealthyRenegade.com to learn how to reduce stress by creating a preaching calendar.)

Over the last decade, this reactive health lifestyle has resulted in fifty pounds of unwanted weight, knee pain, high blood pressure and not a few bouts of depression. Alex never planned to get into a position where his health compromised his ability to fulfill the potential God put within him; the problem was, he never planned not to.

Rob Renegade, on the other hand, adopted a different mindset about his health many years ago. Looking around and seeing his fellow pastors struggling with weight, illness and stress, he decided to walk a different path. He began to understand that if he wanted to be fit to serve for as long as possible, he needed to start cooperating with his creator to keep his body ready for the task. So, Rob made some simple changes. He became more mindful about his eating habits; he became intentional about working more physical activity into his days; and he started proactively managing his rest and his stress levels. Now well into middle age, he has more energy and vigor to fulfill his calling than he did when he first graduated from seminary. His health has become a tool that works for him rather than an obstacle that keeps him from God's best.

Average vs. Renegade

In his classic spoken word recording *Lead the Field*, Earl Nightingale said, "If you want to be successful in life and you have no role models, look at what the majority of people are doing and do the opposite. The majority is always wrong."[6] When it comes to being a pastor, I couldn't agree more. If you want to grow a healthy church and have a happy personal life, you cannot do the things an average pastor does (as I discuss in detail in *The Renegade Pastor: Abandoning Average in Your Life and Ministry* and in my ongoing Renegade Pastors coaching network. For more information, go to HealthyRenegade.com). The same truth applies to your health. If you want to live a life full of the physical vitality you need in order to be able to do all that God has called you to, then you must decide to go renegade with your health. In other words, commit to being a healthy renegade pastor.

> Are you ready to live a life full of the physical vitality you need to be able to do all that God has called you to? Time to go renegade.

A renegade is someone who has abandoned average in favor of excellence; someone who rises up against resistance, mediocrity and conformity. He's not contrarian for contrarian's sake. He's not looking for a fight with other people, but with the devil himself. He's not critical or cynical, but analytical in his thinking about what works and what doesn't. A renegade pastor is obedient to the word of God and passionately abandoned for the kingdom. He has made a decision to step out of the status quo and get back to the business of reflecting God's glory in every single aspect of his life.

On an individual level, the renegade pastor is someone who lives in a state of faithful pro-activity. The renegade's church is healthy and growing, as is he. The renegade pastor is a hard worker, but he knows how to work efficiently and manage his time for maximum benefit, avoiding unnecessary stress and all of its negative effects. He has quality relationships in his life. He is intentional about keeping his body—his most critical tool for ministry on this earth—healthy and strong. He knows how to identify godly health goals and pursue them. And, unlike the average pastor, the renegade has peace about his health, his work and his future. He experiences the fulfillment that comes with embracing the life God has called him to.

The Renegade Pastor - Defining Characteristics -
• Abandons average
• Challenges status quo thinking
• Lives a pro-active lifestyle
• Stands against resistance and mediocrity
• Remains healthy and full of energy
• Passionately abandoned to the will of God
• Dedicates time to rest and growth
• Experiences fulfillment

VERSUS
The Average Pastor
- Defining Characteristics -

- Frustrated
- Overweight
- Short on time
- Low on energy
- Dealing with chronic, lifestyle-related health issues
- Lives a reactive life
- Unable to say 'yes' to God's purposes
- Not experiencing fulfillment

The differences between an average pastor and a renegade pastor are strikingly clear. So the question then becomes: *Do you want to be average or do you want to be renegade?* And if you are ready to go renegade, how do you bridge the divide between these two dichotomies? What can you do to develop a lifestyle that look less like Alex's and more like Rob's? The answers lie in the pages ahead. (For more insight into what distinguishes a renegade pastor from an average pastor, including a list of the Seven Commitments of a Renegade Pastor, visit HealthyRenegade.com.)

. . .

2

Abandoning Average:
Get Unstuck

Though no one can go back and make a brand new start,
anyone can start from now and make a brand new ending.
CARL BARD

Therefore, since we are surrounded by such a huge crowd of
witnesses to the life of faith, let us strip off every weight that slows us down,
especially the sin that so easily trips us up. And let us run with endurance
the race God has set before us. We do this by keeping our eyes on Jesus,
the champion who initiates and perfects our faith.
HEBREWS 12:1-2

Are you stuck in a rut? That's how Alex Average feels most of the time. Maybe you can relate to a typical day for him. See if this sounds familiar: You get up early and check your messages and emails, only to find that there is a problem waiting for you that has to be dealt with immediately. Once you put out that early morning fire, you take a quick shower and kiss your family goodbye while you are stuffing some breakfast into your mouth. There's no time to spare; you are already late for your first appointment. You fight traffic to get to work and settle in for a long, hard day.

After you leave the office (later than you intended to, of course), you swing by the hospital to encourage a sick church member.

Starving, you grab a snack from the hospital vending machine to tide you over. Traffic is a mess and you get home frazzled. You eat a quick, not-so-healthy dinner and spend a little time with your family. Once everyone is in bed, you regroup and put a few more hours of work in. When you finally get to bed yourself, you lay awake thinking about issues in the church and mentally preparing to-do lists for the next day. The following morning, the alarm goes off bright and early. You drag out of bed and do it all over again.

Your present does not have to equal your future.

Maybe you have grand visions in the corners of your mind about losing some weight and getting healthier. But as the days continue to roll by, your plans for eating better, resting more and exercising get pushed further and further down the priority list. Like Alex—like most average pastors—you feel stuck. You are practicing a lifestyle that has predictable health consequences, but you don't have the time or energy to break the cycle.

Here's some great news: your present does not have to equal your future. No matter your current state of being, you can get unstuck and move toward living the life of excellence God has called you to. Change is possible. Both of us (Nelson and Steve) used to be right where you are, but with some key decisions, intentional action and a lot of grace, we were both able to break out of unhealthy lifestyle ruts and start living as renegades in passionate pursuit of God's purposes. Here are our stories.

Steve's Story

My weight problem started as a child. I (Steve) was more than just a little husky. I was fat. I weighed one hundred pounds in the first grade, which was incredibly unusual in 1963. Unfortunately, I had started developing bad eating habits almost as early as I began eating. Most of the food I ate was either fried or loaded with sugar. The only thing that saved me from debilitating childhood obesity was my love of sports. I got involved with football at an early age and ended up being good at it. So, even though my diet left a lot to be desired, I was able to keep my weight somewhat in check thanks to my activity on the football field.

Football also gave me the chance to go to college. While several small schools wanted to recruit me, I ended up accepting a full scholarship to Liberty University. Stepping onto Liberty's campus as a freshman, I assumed that I would eventually become a coach or maybe a businessman. However, shortly into my first year, I felt a clear call from God to go into full-time church ministry. While I loved playing college ball, suddenly I knew that nothing other than pastoring would bring me contentment and joy long-term.

My life at Liberty became consumed with football training, weekend games and doing all I could to prepare to be a pastor. I discussed my call with my girlfriend, Debbie, who later became my wife. We both agreed that we were meant to go into ministry together. We were young, ambitious, energetic and ready to live out our newfound passion.

After graduation, I made a terrible decision—one that would have negative effects on my health, my calling, my ministry, and my personal life. I decided that I was finished with exercise. After over a decade of football drills, cardio conditioning, and weight training, I was tired of the exertion. And I figured that, since my football days were behind me, I didn't have any reason to work out anymore. My new passion, my all-consuming drive, was ministry. I wanted to start a church and I threw myself into the process full-force.

The good news is that the new church began to grow. The bad news is that I began to grow right along with it. Even though I stopped exercising like a college football player, I never stopped eating like one. So I kept growing and growing and growing—until I finally topped out a little over 340 pounds.

Letting my weight get out of control was one of the easiest things I've ever done. People in my church brought me food all the time. If I mentioned that I liked something specific (like Hershey's Milk Chocolate Bars), I would be showered with that very thing. My busy, sporadic schedule led to a lot of fast-food meals. Not to mention, I spent most of my days sitting down. I was either at my desk, in the car, or in meetings. Add in an ongoing addiction to ice cream, which I had to have every night to ease the stress I felt, and I was whipping up a recipe for disaster.

In Galatians 6:7, Paul wrote that if you sow to your flesh, you will reap corruption. That is exactly what I was doing. I was sowing to my flesh by overeating and under-exercising. In the process, I was corrupting the body God had given me. I ended up with three major diseases: high blood pressure (aka the silent killer), high cholesterol, and diabetes. Before I realized it, I was facing a future of medications, doctor's appointments and possibly an early death.

My ministry was growing and prospering. I had a beautiful family who loved me. And I was walking around afraid I would drop dead at any moment, leaving both in distress. The worst part is that, deep down, I knew I was responsible for my condition. I felt humiliated, desperate and alone. I wanted nothing more than to change the reflection in the mirror back to that healthy, vibrant man I used to be.

Today, with intentionality and God's help, I have lost 130 pounds, and have completely reversed my high blood pressure, high cholesterol and diabetes. I am disease free! Plus, out of this experience, God has opened the door for me to create a wonderful ministry called *Losing to Live*. In fact, it was through *Losing to Live* that Nelson and I grew closer, as he was struggling with some of the same challenges.

Before & After

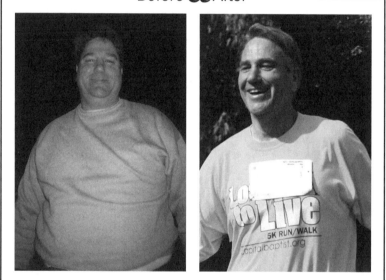

Nelson's Story

A few years ago, I ranked among the millions of people in America who desperately need to embrace a healthier lifestyle. As a church leader, I had spent my entire career building God's kingdom, but in the meantime I had let his temple—my body—fall into disrepair. My physical health just wasn't of much concern to me, even though I had read Paul's words in 1 Corinthians many times:

> *Don't you realize that your body is the temple of the Holy Spirit, who lives in you and was given to you by God? You do not belong to yourself, for God bought you with a high price. So you must honor God with your body.*
> —1 Corinthians 6:19-20

Like most people, I connected these verses with sexual sin and sexual sin only—but they have a much wider implication. I slowly began awakening to the reality that my body is the living, breathing, and walking-around temple of God's spirit. So is yours. And that reality has implications for how we care for ourselves. We are the dwelling place of the Alpha and Omega. Our skin, bones and fleshy guts are home to the Most High. That's a humbling thought, isn't it?

For most of my adult life, I had been able to keep my weight around 185 pounds. Unfortunately, after starting The Journey Church in New York City, that number began to tick up into new territory. I began putting on a few extra pounds every year. Before long, I hit 275. When I saw that number on the scale, I was shocked. I knew I was heavier than usual, but I had no idea I'd let my weight get so out of control.

Even still, the real breaking point didn't come for me until I became a father. After my son was born, I couldn't ignore what I was doing to my body any longer. I remember saying to myself, "I'm not going to be able to chase him around, because I'm so out of shape."

That led me to begin considering everything else my weight and its consequences would keep me from doing in the future, if I didn't make a change. So, I made a decision to take control of my health and then put a definitive plan of action behind that decision.

I started by making simple modifications to my eating habits. Then, I committed to changing myself from being someone who didn't even like to walk very far to becoming someone who could be considered a habitual runner. If you had told me a few years ago that I would start running several times per week and actually enjoy it, I would have called you crazy. But I had left myself little choice. I had to get active. A friend recommended a running program called *Couch to 5K*. As the title implies, the program takes a person who is used to almost no physical activity at all and guides him or her through an incremental process that results in being able to run for thirty minutes without stopping.

The first day I laced up my sneakers and cued up my iPod to give the program a try, I had a hard time running for sixty seconds straight. I remember stumbling back into my New York City apartment—after more walking than running—and saying to my wife, Kelley, "I don't know if I can do this. Maybe it's not for me." But after a day's rest, I tried it again. And then again. And then one more time. And slowly but surely, my endurance began to build. After about eight weeks, I was running for the full thirty minutes. Now, running has become an important part of my life. I miss it when I don't get it in. I'm not saying that I'm always eager to jump into my running shoes. Sometimes I still have to force myself out the door. But even on those days, I always finish my run with a great sense of satisfaction that I am doing my part to keep this body that God gave me in prime working condition.

As they say, the truth will set you free. Thanks to a new perspective on God's plan for my body, my entire mindset toward physical health has shifted. If God has entrusted me with this earthly vessel—not to mention all of the work and plans he has for me while living in it—then where do I get off trashing it by eating what I want and sitting around letting it atrophy? Where do you? How can we stomach treating ourselves so poorly that we can't fully engage in God's purposes for us?

> God wants us to live full, active lives accomplishing the things he put us here to do. We have a responsibility in cooperating with him to make that happen.

Of course, there are a lot of excuses that have become our defense to these types of questions: we have a family history of hearty eaters and big bellies (I loved using that one); we're just big-boned; we don't have time to exercise; and on and on we build our case. All of these excuses—and the hundreds of others we create in a desperate attempt to stay within our carefully constructed comfort zone—keep us from embracing the truth that God wants us to live full, active lives accomplishing the things he put us here to do. We have a responsibility in cooperating with him to make that happen. Life is too short and too precious, and God has invested way too much in us, for us to sit around squandering our potential and letting little things like poor food choices and lack of exercise hold us back from all that he has in store.

Today, I have lost over eighty pounds and completely changed my long-term health trajectory. If I can get the upper hand on my weight and health issues, so can you. You have everything you need to get from where you are to where you want to be. Decide to honor God with your entire being, including the body he has given you. Speaking from the other side of the (ongoing) journey, I can tell you that taking the necessary action to get your physical health under control is more than worth the effort. There's no better gift you can give yourself or those who love you.

Before & After

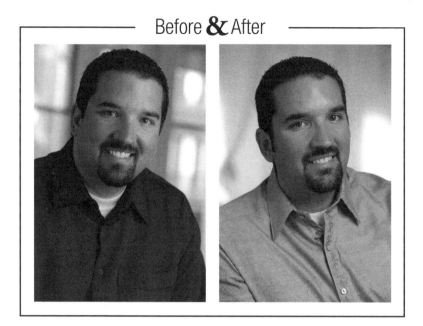

Deciding to Go Renegade

Like both Steve and I, you have to come to a point in your life where you can admit that you are sick and tired of being sick and tired. We were fed up with how we felt, just like you are. We wanted something different for our lives and for our futures, and we want that for you as well. Consider this verse from Isaiah:

> *Do not remember the former things, nor consider the things of old. Behold, I will do a new thing. Now it shall spring forth, shall you not know it? I will even make a road in the wilderness and rivers in the desert.*
> —Isaiah 43:18-19

God says that he will do *a new thing*. Don't dwell on your past. So, you have made some bad health choices. We all have at some point in our lives. God says to forget those things and look ahead to the future.

You may be thinking, "Okay, I went to seminary. These verses don't have anything to do with physical health." Are you sure? God wants to do a new thing in every single one of us *in* and *through* Jesus Christ. He is an *unstuck* kind of God. During his ministry on earth, Jesus constantly met people where they were, forgave them, helped them break free from their current circumstances, and showed them a new way to live. He wants to do the same for you, in every way—even, and maybe especially, in your physical health. Are you ready?

· · ·

Healthy Renegade Pastor Profile

Ben Emmons
South County Church, Lorton, VA

I am thirty-seven years old and have had the honor of serving God in full-time ministry for thirteen years. I have always struggled with eating a lot of unhealthy food. For me, being a pastor did not encourage an inactive and unhealthy lifestyle; it simply supported the one I already had. I was unhealthy and overweight for the first six years of my ministry. It was a sad day when I had to face the fact that I had let myself get to the point of weighing 321 pounds.

In 2007, the Holy Spirit convicted me for not practicing what I was preaching. I came to realize that I lacked self-control and discipline. I believe the Lord was telling me that I would die at a young age, leaving my wife without a husband and my children without a father, if I didn't change things in my life. This was a wake up call for me. I immediately began living according to my new conviction that I needed to honor God by caring for my physical body. Over the next year, I lost 131 pounds, and for the first time I experienced the abundant life that Jesus described in John 10:10.

This transformation was not easy. I was addicted to food. I have always had a huge sweet tooth, so for me avoiding unhealthy foods has always been difficult. I was and still am tempted to be a stress eater. When things got out of control in my life or I was overly stressed, I misled myself into believing that food was the answer to my problems and anxiety. It was not until I went through this lifestyle change that I learned to fully trust God and stop looking to the pantry to solve my problems.

Being a pastor in full-time ministry can certainly make living healthy and making good food choices more difficult. As pastors, I believe we have bought into the cultural philosophy that accepts, and even seems to encourage, overweight spiritual leaders. There is always food at our church activities, gatherings, and small groups, and my church has a great spread of food (healthy and unhealthy) on Sunday mornings at our main church services. It seems like church life centers around eating. Let's be honest, something special happens when you eat together.

However, at our church we have begun to break the cycle of unhealthy eating. Instead of doing away with eating altogether or going 100% donut-less, we make sure we have healthy options available. Some examples of these healthy options are fresh fruit, oatmeal, vegetables, and hard-boiled eggs. Our church has an amazing hospitality team and it seems like they are always going out of their way to include as many healthy options as possible for our people.

I am thrilled to tell you that all of my hard work and dedication to changing my life and health has paid off tremendously. I have gone from not being able to run a quarter of a mile in 2007 to running seven marathons, countless half marathons and participating in two half ironmen competitions. I am no Ironman world champion or Olympic gold medalist runner, but I am happy to report that I am in the best shape of my life. As of the date of this writing, I am celebrating my 2000th consecutive day of running at a least a mile. That's a huge change for me!

I believe that getting people moving is so important. We started a group at our church called the South County Movers, which currently has about forty people in it who gather each Saturday to walk, run, or crawl depending on their physical abilities. Typically, we exercise together for about an hour every week. The best part is that we encourage accountability for improved physical health.

I am constantly reminding my church that honoring God by caring for their physical health is critical and biblical. I talk with my people about how their food choices are important to God and to his design for their futures, and about the fact that they need to care for His dwelling place and build their strength to serve him with greater efficiency. In reality, everything we do can be brought back to the idea that God cares about our health holistically. The designer cares about the design.

Eating healthy and exercising is just the way I do life now. Every day, my goal is to honor God with my nutrition and through physical exercise. I changed my life and you can too! God wants you to be healthy, and I have a feeling that you want to be healthy as well. What's stopping you?

Ben's Advice: Balance, boundaries and healthy habits are critical for future success. It is okay to say no!

Before & After

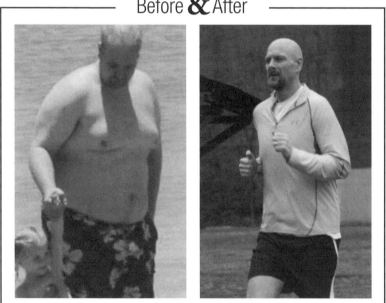

3

Abandoning Average:
Surrender Your Body to God

The reason why many are still troubled, still seeking, still making little forward progress is because they haven't yet come to the end of themselves. We're still trying to give orders, and interfering with God's work within us.

A.W. TOZER

Don't you realize that your body is the temple of the Holy Spirit, who lives in you and was given to you by God? You do not belong to yourself, for God bought you with a high price. So you must honor God with your body.

1 CORINTHIANS 6:19-20

As a teenager, I spent some time traveling and speaking at young entrepreneur conferences around the country. Thanks to that circuit, I had the privilege of working alongside the late Zig Ziglar. A great businessman and leader, Zig spoke eloquently about matters of vision, change, work and commitment. One statement Zig used to make often that has stuck with me through the years was this: "It's character that got us out of bed, commitment that moved us to action, and discipline that enabled us to follow through."

Character, commitment and discipline—the ability to move from where you are to where you want to be will flow from these three things. All intentional change is birthed out of character, anchored in the commitments you make and executed through discipline. Your character drove you to pick up this book because something within you is longing to take your health up a notch—to the level where you know it should be. Perhaps you can feel weight, stress and sickness tugging at your shirtsleeve, and you know it's leading you down a path to be avoided at all costs.

Discipline will determine how well you follow through with the adjustments you want and need to make. In the pages ahead, I will give you much of the knowledge and tools you need to begin living like a healthy renegade, but how well you apply them is completely up to you. No one else can change your life for you. I can guarantee, though, if you will make a decision to raise your game for God's glory, he will meet you in that place and help you get to where he wants you to be.

That leaves the issue of commitments. The commitments you choose to make in your life will determine your path through this world. If you look back through your past, I'm sure you can identify a handful of commitments that have had a major impact on where you are today. You made a commitment to give your life to God and follow him into the work of ministry. Maybe you made a commitment to go to one particular school over another and that commitment put you on your current trajectory. You may have made the commitment to share your life with a spouse, or you may still be hoping to make that commitment one day. If you have children, you've made a commitment to care for them and raise them well. Each one of these is a life-changing commitment.

Getting your health on track is also a life-changing commitment. When you have your body under control, you are free to pursue God's plans for you, unburdened by the very thing that drags so many people down into an average, mundane existence. It's hard to get excited about the future when you don't feel well; it's not easy to shine the light of the gospel when you're struggling to get through every day. But if you will commit to making your health a priority and then follow that commitment up with simple (note that I said simple, not necessarily easy) lifestyle changes, you can transform your health and revolutionize your ability to interact in the world in a way that brings God the most glory. The first step is to surrender your body to the one who created it.

Full Surrender

When I (Steve) hit the crisis point in my life, I knew I needed to do something but I didn't know exactly what that something should be. There's so much contradicting information out there about the healthiest and most effective ways to get in shape. A quick web search leads to dozens of companies selling tempting shortcuts and promoting "experts" who will do nothing but tell you what you want to hear to get you on their weight loss program. As I prayed about how to get started, James' words about wisdom kept coming to me:

If you need wisdom, ask our generous God,
and he will give it to you.
—James 1:5

Instead of looking to outside sources, I decided to start my journey by going to the ultimate source—the Bible. After all, since God is the one who created my body and yours, it only makes sense that he would have something to say about how we should take care of them, right? I started by searching the Bible for verses mentioning the word *body*. Believe it or not, there are close to 200 verses that include the word. Now, of course, some of them are talking about the body of Christ, or about our glorified bodies in heaven, but most of the references deal with how we should view and treat the bodies we have on this earth.

As I studied each verse, new truths jumped out at me. Scripture I'd heard my whole life began to resonate in an entirely new way. Of course I knew that my body was made *by* God, but I hadn't really considered the fact that it was also made *for* God:

[Our bodies] **were made for the Lord,**
and the Lord cares about our bodies.
—1 Corinthians 6:13 (emphasis added)

If our bodies are made for the Lord and he cares about them, shouldn't we care about them too? I have spent years preaching about the importance of surrendering your entire being to God, but all the while, I had a major blind spot. In my mind, surrendering myself didn't mean surrendering my ice cream spoon. It didn't mean surrendering my unwillingness to exercise. When I thought about my physical health at all, I assumed it was mine to manage (read: squander) as I pleased. But through prayer and study, God began to impress a new realization on me: My body wasn't created for my own gratification, but for his glory.

In the past, there had been a disconnect between my belief system and my behavior. Even though I believed Paul's assertion that my body was the temple of God, I chose to think of that temple in terms of purely spiritual implications. When I did apply the verse to physicality, I thought mostly of sexual purity, as mentioned, or of not becoming consumed with addictive vices that could harm me. However, the whole time I was standing in the pulpit preaching on the importance of keeping the temple pure, I may as well have had gravy dripping down my double chin and running off of my bulging belly. I was in such bad physical shape that after three services on Sunday morning, I was ready to pass out. I was a hypocrite; I was a temple trasher. I was treating my body like it didn't matter—and enjoying every minute.

Your body wasn't created for your own gratification, but for God's glory.

Thankfully, I became broken enough to admit that I wasn't living out God's best plan for my physical wellbeing. He had more in store for my body than I had been choosing to see; he wanted to use it as a tool to do his work in the world and my poor decisions were hindering those purposes. Talk about convicting!

The Bible is clear that our bodies were created to glorify the Creator. Obesity, diabetes, high blood pressure, high cholesterol and other lifestyle-induced health conditions don't do much to glorify God. They don't shine his excellence and the abundant life he offers to an on-looking world—far from it. We are called to do so much better.

> Our bodies were created to glorify the Creator.

Good Health = Good Stewardship

When I talk to people about tithing, one of the first truths I make sure they understand is that their money is not their own anyway. It belongs to God; they have just been trusted to manage it well. They have been appointed stewards of what they've been given.

The same holds true for your body and mine. Your body is not your own. The one who created it has simply entrusted it to you for a period of time. You are called to steward your health in the same way you steward your money, your time, and your relationships—and that stewardship is not optional. As Rick Warren wrote in *The Daniel Plan*:

> *This life is preparation for our next life, which will last forever in eternity. God is testing you on earth to see what he can trust you with in eternity. He is watching how you use your time, your money, your talents, your opportunities, your mind, and yes, even your body. Are you making the most of what you've been given? God isn't going to evaluate you on the basis of the bodies he gave to other people, but he will judge what you did with what you have been given.[1]*

Have you ever thought about having to stand before God and give an account for how you've cared for your body—for how well you've eaten, how active you've been in an effort to stay healthy, how intentional you've been about managing your stress levels to avoid negative health consequences? That's a scary notion, isn't it? Most of us have never thought that deeply about our physical stewardship responsibility. The good news is that it's not too late to start. It's not too late to surrender your body—to surrender every aspect of your physical health and wellbeing—to God.

Before you begin any directed plan to get yourself in better shape, take time to pray. Talk with God about your current physical condition. If you've been a temple trasher too, repent of that. Ask him to help you be a good steward of the earthly vessel he has entrusted to you. Only then, working from the foundational understanding that your body is not your own but his, can you forge ahead into the realm of the healthy renegades.

. . .

Healthy Renegade Pastor Profile

Don Ross
Creekside Church, Mountlake Terrace, WA

I am fifty-eight years old and have been in ministry for forty years. I have struggled with maintaining a healthy weight since college. In the past, I have tried just about every program out there, and each one helped in some small way. However, I always wanted the program to do the work for me. My problem was that I never took personal responsibility for my results. Not only was I an emotional eater, I also ate to medicate pain. As a Christian, I didn't drink or do drugs, so food became my default vice. I also struggled with regular exercise and portion control.

When I started this journey, I weighed 267 pounds. To date, I have lost a total of thirty-eight pounds, and have twenty-five more to go. I am not going to use ministry as an excuse, but it's true that people often want to meet in restaurants. No one put a gun to my head and made me order the food I was eating, but the environment made things hard for me—that is, before I gave control of my eating to Jesus. After that, it really didn't matter where I met people. I was able to control my eating habits.

The first time I read Steve's book, *Bod4God: The Four Keys to Weight Loss*, I cried my way through it because I finally had some hope from a spiritual point of view. I always knew my weight was a spiritual problem at the root, but *Bod4God* drove that home. I copied every scripture in the book (and there are a lot of them) to help renew my mind.

I became so excited about my new lifestyle and what it did for me, that I brought it to my church. It has made a huge impact; so far we have lost over 2,500 pounds collectively. Fat Christians make a public statement that they are undisciplined. An undisciplined person is often an untrustworthy person. This means that our personal lives and how we take care of our bodies impacts how we carry the gospel. Also, not taking care of ourselves well shortens how many years we can serve the message of the gospel here on earth. Now, I preach about what the Bible says about health during our annual stewardship series. I talk about the stewardship of our bodies in areas such as sex, eating and rest.

I have found that it is easier for me to eat right than to commit to exercising regularly. Exercising with my wife is helpful, and it has helped her lose fifty pounds as well. I am very proud of her. We make a great team, and we are getting healthier together. Don't try to do this alone; be accountable to someone and decide to exercise together.

If you are overweight like I was and struggling in this area, don't let the idolatry of food shorten your ability to impact others with the gospel because you are not around anymore. I only wish I had been obedient to Jesus sooner. It is time for pastors to wake up and start producing change in themselves and in their churches.

Don's Advice: Get a handle on eating and exercise now. Give Jesus control of your body and save your life.

Before & After

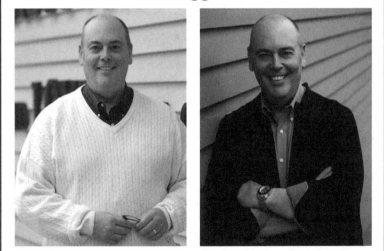

4

Abandoning Average:
Stop Making Excuses

Ninety-nine percent of failures come from people who
have the habit of making excuses.
GEORGE WASHINGTON

Don't copy the behavior and customs of this world, but let God transform you into
a new person by changing the way you think. Then you will learn to know God's
will for you, which is good and pleasing and perfect.
ROMANS 12:2

Excuses, excuses, excuses! I've heard them all as I've worked with
people across the country to get healthy. I hate excuses, but I can
tell you who loves them—Satan. The enemy of your soul loves using
carefully crafted excuses to cast doubt over the best of intentions. Just
think about this: if you are stuck in the rut of average—unhealthy,
not living the abundant life in Christ and not working to your full
potential as a church leader—then the enemy is thrilled. He's getting
his exercise doing a happy dance because you are compromised; you
are not being as effective for the kingdom as you could be.

You know as well as I do that spiritual warfare is nothing to be
taken lightly. What you may not realize is that your health is not
exempt from the war. Satan will do anything he can to throw up
roadblocks to your ability to live the life God has in store for you,

and getting you to sabotage your own body is one of his most cunning tactics. As Jesus said:

> *The thief's purpose is to steal and kill and destroy.*
> *My purpose is to give them a rich and satisfying life.*
> —John 10:10

If Satan can steal your health, kill your drive and destroy your peace of mind, then your ability to do God's work well will be obliterated. Thankfully, there are things you can do to keep the enemy's schemes at bay. Start by surrendering your body to God, as we discussed in the last chapter. Then, stop making excuses.

The Most Common Excuses

When you make excuses for your weight or your poor health, you are reinforcing the very lies Satan wants you to believe. Those lies can be so subtle that you probably don't even realize they are coming from him. You may have even grown up hearing them spoken over you, so you have accepted them as reality without giving a second thought to their true source.

Surprisingly, Satan isn't that creative in the excuses he feeds you and me. He doesn't have to be. Most of us are all too willing to latch on to the first excuse we can find to justify why our weight or our illness is beyond our control. Here are a few of the most common ones I've heard over the years:

- *I'm just big boned.*

- *I'm Italian/German/Irish/(pick a nationality)—*
  I'm supposed to be fat.

- *I don't like the taste of healthy foods.*

- *Obesity/diabetes/heart disease runs in my family. It must*
  be genetic.

That last one reminds me of a joke I heard recently: An overweight man goes to his family doctor for a checkup. When the doctor expresses concern over his weight, the man says, "Doc, the problem is that obesity runs in my family." To which the doctor replies, "No, the problem is that no one in your family runs!"

When you cut through all of the smoke screens and trick mirrors people use to justify their poor choices and bad behavior, most of the excuses out there can be filed under two main categories: *I don't have time* and *I'm too tired.* Let's examine what really lies beneath each of these:

I don't have time—A lack of time is the number one excuse people offer up for neglecting their health. Unfortunately for the excuse makers, it's never a valid claim. Now, don't misunderstand me. I know that we are all overwhelmingly busy. There's always something else on the to-do list that has to be taken care of right away. But I would suggest to you that, no matter how busy your life is, you will always find time for what you consider to be most important.

Do you have time to get quiet before God each day? Do you have time to spend with your kids? Do you have time to connect with your staff about the weekend service? Of course you do, because you understand the importance of those things. When you understand the importance of being proactive about your health—and hopefully that won't be at the point of a life or death crisis for you—you will find the time to do it. Period. It's not a question of time; it's a question of priorities.

Still, those of us working in the ministry love the time excuse because it sounds so self-sacrificial. It allows us to play the holy victim. Part of our calling is to care for the needs of others. So, when we don't have time to eat well or work out because we are busy serving other people, well, that's just the price we pay for doing God's work, right? Wrong. This is nothing more than a righteous-sounding reason for taking our temple for granted.

In reality, failing to take the time to eat well and exercise today means that more of your time will be occupied by health concerns tomorrow. Waiting for doctor's appointments, having prescriptions filled and continuously checking your sugar levels and blood pressure take a lot of time out of your busy schedule. Those are precious hours spent away from your family and your ministry. Better to make time for healthy living now than to be forced to spend time (and money) dealing with health problems down the road.

Once I committed to making exercise and healthy eating part of my routine, I became addicted to the results. What it does for me physically, mentally, emotionally, and spiritually is hard to overstate. Thanks to prioritizing my health, I'm now more efficient with my time and better able to help all of the other people I had been using as an excuse. I have a clearer mind and more energy to tackle every day's work. Healthy living is truly an investment of time rather than an expenditure—one that seems to multiply the hours exponentially. (Discover proven time management principles you can start applying right away at HealthyRenegade.com.)

I'm too tired—Poor food choices combined with a lack of physical activity are a recipe for constant lethargy, which makes this one a self-perpetuating excuse. If you are inclined to play the tired card, remember: the biggest reason you are so tired is because of your unhealthy lifestyle. The longer you subsist in this kind of lifestyle, the more tired you are going to be—which will make the excuse even harder to break free from. The only answer is to be intentional about taking a first step toward health. Make a healthy meal even though you are tired. Go for a walk even if you don't feel like it. Over time, with consistent effort, you will have more and more energy and this excuse will begin to evaporate.

Shifting Focus

Excuses are a natural byproduct of wrong focus. They are the result of concentrating on the obstacles to a healthy lifestyle—and, believe me, there will be plenty of legitimate obstacles to concentrate on if you want to—rather than on the opportunities good health provides. Instead of bemoaning how hard it will be to change your bad habits, shift your attention to all of the ways that being healthy will transform your life for the better. When you have a big enough *why*, the *how* won't seem so intimidating. Here are just three of the benefits a healthy lifestyle provides:

1. *Good health will help you maximize your life.* Since God went to such lengths to design the intricate details of your body (Psalm 139), you should want to maximize what he can do through it while you are alive. When you run it down with unhealthy foods, lack of exercise, and massive doses of stress, you block that opportunity. Rather than maximizing your life, you trade it in for a counterfeit version of God's best. Poor health choices will limit your potential and likely shorten the length of your days on this earth, but taking care of yourself will open the door to being able to fully engage in the abundant life God has in store for you.

2. *Good health will help you feel better and be more productive each day.* When you get your health on track, you will have more energy every day. You will have fewer aches and pains. Your mind will be clearer. You will look better and be happier. You will be able to work harder and connect with the people in your life with more enthusiasm. Doesn't that sound like a great way to live? Don't let excuses rob you of your opportunity to live the life you were created for.

3. *Good health gives you a new opportunity to worship God.*
    Since your body is the temple of God (1 Corinthians
    6:1920), taking care of that temple is a form of worship.
    Intentional good health brings God glory. Again, you
    and I are called to honor God by reflecting his excellence
    in every way—including with our physical wellbeing.
    Don't miss the opportunity you have to worship your
    Heavenly Father and show his excellence to the world by
    being an example of refreshing, vibrant health.

> Don't let excuses rob you of your opportunity to live the
> life you were created for.

• • •

Healthy Renegade Pastor Profile

Gary Moritz
Twin City Baptist Church, Lunenburg, MA

I am forty years old, have been in full-time ministry for thirteen years, and am 100% sold out to my Papa...God! However, I didn't realize as a young pastor just starting out, that my other papa, Papa John's Pizza, was going to contribute to a forty-pound weight gain during my first few years of ministry. This was a shock for me since I entered the ministry right after leaving the United States Marine Corps.

Dealing with the demands of being a pastor is not easy, and I found that I was more consumed with reaching and ministering to people than I was with maintaining a healthy weight and lifestyle. My wake-up call came when my doctor looked at me and said that my cholesterol was sky high and that I was at a higher risk of having a heart attack based on my family history, weight and eating/exercising habits. I knew I had to act fast. My wife and I were new parents. For the sake of my family, I needed to make some changes.

One of the biggest struggles I faced as a pastor was trying to get my schedule to jive with living healthier. I worked long hours and seemed to be in meeting after meeting. I found that it took a lot more planning to eat fresh, healthy and organic than it did to rush through the drive-thru of a fast food joint. Even though it hadn't taken me long after leaving the military to revert back to my Italian roots where pizza and pasta were a food group, I was determined to get my health back, so I started making changes in my life. I started to form new habits, and all of the hard work started to pay off. Praise God, I was able to lose about thirty-three pounds. I kicked the cannolis and created a healthy lifestyle in Christ.

Today, I make it a point to have a good balanced breakfast before I leave home, and I prioritize my time in the gym by actually adding it to my calendar. Basically, I book an appointment with myself to exercise. One of the turning points for me was when I started viewing food as fuel and water as a fuel injection for my body. Like many pastors, I used to drink coffee all day. I had to learn to fight the urge to pull in to my favorite coffee shop and instead drink from the water bottle I filled up at home.

Gluttony is a sin, and we need to continually caution our people on the dangers of it. I am constantly reminding people of what I call the most powerful law in the universe: the law found in Galatians 6:7, where God talks about sowing and reaping. If we get this law working for good in our life, great things will happen; however, if we are sowing to our flesh, the Bible promises that we will reap corruption.

Remember, our lives as pastors speak volumes! People are watching how we live and how we act. They will notice our big bellies before our big Bibles. They are even watching what we eat. Set a good example for the people you lead. Be healthy.

Gary's Advice: Don't make pizza your communion wafer!

Before & After

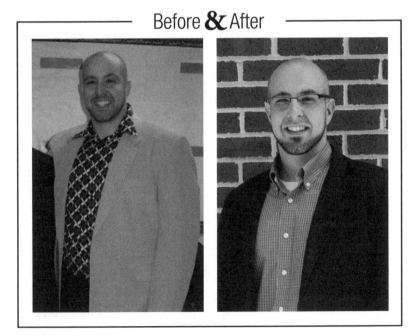

5

Abandoning Average:
Start Making Changes

If you do what you've always done, you'll get what you've always gotten.
TONY ROBBINS

Since, then, we do not have the excuse of ignorance, everything—
and I do mean everything—connected with that old way of life has to go.
It's rotten through and through. Get rid of it! And then take on an entirely
new way of life—a God-fashioned life, a life renewed from the inside and working
itself into your conduct as God accurately reproduces his character in you.
EPHESIANS 4:22-24 (MSG)

One of my mentors used to say, "There is no elevator to success. You have to take the stairs." When it comes to physical health, there are plenty of people out there buying into elevator philosophies— pills, powders, fad diets, extreme exercise plans... you name it. Why? Because making an ongoing lifestyle change sounds a little too much like taking the stairs. It will probably even require walking some literal ones! Something within us wants to opt for the quick fix. But quick fixes always lead to short-term results, followed by a face plant right back into the condition we were in before we started.

Think, for example, about the many popular diets that advocate losing weight by cutting out carbohydrates. Sure, that elevator will take you to a skinnier floor, but only as long as you stay on it. The problem is that eschewing carbohydrates for life isn't only unrealistic, it's not a nutritionally sound approach to health. Your body needs good carbohydrates to function effectively (as we'll see in chapter 8). As soon as you start eating them again, the weight returns with a vengeance and you are back on the ground level, if not in the basement. Health-related shortcuts will only put you further behind in the long run. The only way to get and stay physically well is to commit to an ongoing healthy, balanced lifestyle.

An Original Renegade

As I began my journey toward health, I found myself particularly interested in studying the life of Moses. Moses was the leader of over a million people, serving as a counselor, an advocate, and a judge. He led a life of vision and momentum, leaving a legacy that still lives on thousands of years after his death. Talk about someone who abandoned average in passionate pursuit of God's plans! Moses was one of the original renegades.

Moses wasn't only renegade when it came to his ministry; he was also renegade in his approach to health. Look how he is described at the end of his life:

> *Moses was 120 years old when he died, yet his eyesight was*
> *clear, and he was as strong as ever.*
> —Deuteronomy 34:7

Moses was *strong as ever* at 120 years old, while most of us feel the wear and tear of age by our early forties. Of course, we live in a different time than Moses, but we can draw some pretty accurate conclusions as to how he took care of himself from what scripture tells us about his lifestyle. We know he stayed active by walking a lot (as documented throughout Exodus), he ate only the portion of food that had been provided for him each given day (Exodus 16:4), and he communed intimately with God (Exodus 33:11).

As I am getting older, I have developed a passion to live a long life. I want to live to be at least a hundred years old, just like Moses. But I don't just want to suck air until I'm a hundred; I want to be healthy, strong and productive until my last day. I want to make a difference with my life and impact others for as long as possible. Just like Moses, I want to honor God with the health choices I make so I can experience the full measure of what he has for me. How about you?

Moses adhered to a lifestyle that, along with God's help and grace, allowed him to live to a vibrant old age. In order to become a healthy renegade, you also have to adopt a lifestyle of health—one that honors God and that he can honor in return; one that sows seeds of physical vitality and strength rather than seeds of sloth and sickness. To get there, focus on making ongoing lifestyle changes in four areas:

1. How you **eat**.
2. How much you **move**.
3. How well you **rest**.
4. How you **handle stress**.

In the pages ahead, we'll dig into the keys to making sustainable lifestyle changes and achieving health in each of these areas. Here's a quick overview of each one:

Eating—To begin eating for life, you have to do two primary things—eat smaller quantities and focus on foods that will give your body the nutrition it craves. In the Bible, God gives specific instructions for the types of food he created to keep our bodies thriving. Unfortunately, you and I have largely traded his diet advice for nutritionally defunct helpings of speed and convenience. Worse, the foods most of us have trained our bodies to love are the very foods that keep us slaves to excess weight, inflammation, and chronic illnesses. Getting healthy means moving away from food choices that lead only to temporary pleasure and ultimately to death, back toward life-giving nutrition.

Moving—We were made to move, but given the nature of our work most of us spend our days sitting down. This is more dangerous than you may think. Current research shows that physical inactivity significantly raises the risk of heart disease, cancer and obesity. A sedentary lifestyle is the new smoking. But don't worry—there are ways to work regular exercise and more overall movement into your life without having to become an Olympic athlete. Small, simple changes in how you move your body can go a long way.

Resting—How much sleep did you get last night? Did you take a Sabbath last week or did you feel like you couldn't afford to? (For a powerful resource on the power of the Sabbath, including a thirty-minute Q&A session, visit HealthyRenegade.com.) Rest is critically important to keeping you and me healthy now and in years to come, but we always tend to think we can get by with a little less of it. We like to pat ourselves on the back if we sleep less than the next guy; it makes us feel like we are more hard-core, more productive—but that's a fallacy. There is nothing positive about giving up sleep in the name of getting more done; usually the approach backfires anyway. We end up getting less done because we aren't as alert or focused as we would've been if we'd allowed our bodies to rest properly. Not to mention, lack of sleep leads to a whole host of physical downfalls over time. To become a healthy renegade, you have to start resting like one.

Renewing—Chronic stress is as detrimental to your physical health as deep-fried foods, couch sitting and lack of sleep. It raises cortisol levels in your blood, which leads to a weakened immune system and a wide range of chronic physical conditions. Learning to manage stress well is essential to being healthy—and this goes far beyond issues of time management and delegation. Instead of thinking about how to squeeze more into your day, ask yourself if you are harboring resentment against someone. Do you have a bad attitude about a situation you are facing? Questions like these can give you a clue to the state of your emotional wellbeing. If you want to live a healthy life, you have to make sure your heart and mind are at peace no matter what's going on around you. (Go to HealthyRenegade.com to download *Managing the Stress of Ministry*—a free audio resource on how to manage stress well and become a more a more effective pastor.)

Small Steps to Life

Incremental steps are the key in moving from an unhealthy lifestyle to one that will serve you and those around you well. Don't think you have to undergo a sudden extreme makeover in order to get where you need to be. Rather, focus on minor improvements every day, every week, and every month. Over time, you'll be amazed at the cumulative effect of your small efforts.

> Success is the sum of small efforts, repeated day in and day out. —Robert Collier

What if you could improve your health by just 10% over the next six months? What if you could improve it by 10% more the following six? That would make you 20% healthier this time next year than you are right now. If you could do that again the following year, you'd be 40% healthier two years from now. Small changes to your lifestyle can get you there. You don't have to be intimidated by anything discussed in the pages ahead. Just take in what works for you and make the changes that will help you get to where you know you need to be.

Throughout the rest of the book, at the end of each chapter, I will be suggesting *Small Steps to Life* that can help you begin making simple changes that will lead to great rewards. A small step for you might be to start cutting out fast food or pulling the skin off of your fried chicken. Maybe you decide to follow the old advice and eat an apple every day. Or you commit to drinking one bottle of water each day and cutting out one soda. These are small steps that will work together over time to revolutionize your health, taking you from feeling fat, sick and average back to being on fire for all that God wants to do in you and through you until he calls you home.

. . .

Healthy Renegade Pastor Profile

Chuck Hildbold
Jennerstown United Methodist Church, Jennerstown, PA

I am fifty-seven years old and have been in ministry for thirty-five years. I have been struggling with my weight and maintaining a healthy lifestyle for about fifteen of those years. I have always found it somewhat enjoyable to be active and when I am, not only am I in a better mood but I'm also more effective as a husband, father and pastor.

I used to wrestle and play a lot of softball, which kept me in fairly good physical shape. However, as I got older and the demands of ministry increased, I found myself being less and less active because it was hard to find the time. My eating habits also declined considerably. I would eat late at night or while working, even if I didn't really need to.

I am excited to share with you that I have lost twenty-six pounds since I started making health and wellness a priority in my life. But this weight loss did not happen by chance. I had to make time for the changes that needed to be made.

Living a healthy lifestyle is a great way to witness to others. Our United Methodist Church has many obese pastors who need help desperately. Personally, I would have a very difficult time admiring someone or following someone who preaches to me about giving thanks for the bodies God has given us when they are grossly overweight or not taking care of their own body. I am training my congregation to understand that our bodies are the temple of the Holy Spirit, that we are made in God's image and that we are his crowning jewel. I want to honor God with what he has given to me, and I want my congregation to do the same.

That is why I make it a priority to balance eating right and exercising with the difficult demands of ministry. I have created a daily routine to support that. I get up in the morning and write a devotional while my son gets ready for school. After he leaves, I do one of three things: I either do an intense ten-minute workout involving cardio, core and stretching, or a twenty to thirty minute jaunt on the elliptical, or I walk outside with my wife for thirty minutes.

If you are struggling with your health and weight, set a schedule that includes work as well as exercise. Make it a point to eat at a regular time and not when you happen to get home late at night after meetings. Even if you don't think weight is going to be a problem for you, as you get older, gravity kicks in and it gets harder to stay trim and healthy. If you are obese see a physician about possible exercise and eating plans.

As a result of becoming a healthy renegade, I am very much aware of the need to honor God with my body. I understand the need to drink more water, which will help make me healthier and avoid ailments later on. I have also changed my eating habits. I used to drink at least a two-liter bottle of Coke every two days. Now, I haven't had soda in over four years. I used to eat a huge bowl of ice cream every night. (After all, it seemed like a basic food group!) But I have curtailed that amount as well.

I want to live as long on this earth as I can for a few reasons. First, I want to live long so that I can spend quality time with my wife, children and grandchildren. Second, so that I can be as effective as possible as a pastor, helping others come to know Jesus and grow closer to him. Third, I want my witness as a dad, husband, pastor and follower of Christ to be evident, not only by the words I say but the way I look and live my life. I want to be and do my best with what God has given to me.

Chuck's Advice: Don't sit around and wonder where that thinner person went! Change your eating habits and get involved in some sort of physical activity.

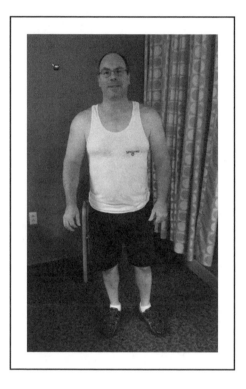

6

Abandoning Average:
Ten Commandments for Healthy Living

Change your opinions, keep to your principles;
change your leaves, keep intact your roots.
VICTOR HUGO

Then Jesus said to his disciples, 'If any of you wants to be my follower,
you must turn from your selfish ways, take up your cross, and follow me.
If you try to hang on to your life, you will lose it. But if you give up
your life for my sake, you will save it.'
MATTHEW 16:24-25

I (Steve) wish someone had sat me down in seminary and talked me through what the Bible has to say about health. But no one did, so I have deciphered a handful of scripture's health principles myself and entitled them the *Ten Commandments for Healthy Living*. These commandments have literally changed my life. They have been the catalyst that has helped me get healthy again, rid myself of disease and trash all the medications I was once on.

Why call them commandments? There are a lot of biblical terms I could have used to describe the principles below. However, I decided to call them commandments within the context of obedience. I was already very familiar with all of the verses these commandments are based on, but I had never really viewed them as imperatives from God; as non-negotiable doctrine that had to be worked into my life in a literal way. You'll be familiar with the following verses too, but like me, you've probably never thought of them in terms of their implications for your health and wellness. Now is the time to begin seeing them through that lens.

Commandment One—Lose to Live

Then Jesus said to his disciples, 'If any of you wants to be my follower, you must turn from your selfish ways, take up your cross, and follow me. If you try to hang on to your life, you will lose it. But if you give up your life for my sake, you will save it.'
—Matthew 16:24-25

Jesus calls you and me to turn from our selfishness and follow him in every area of life. For years, I thought I was doing that. But as I began my journey toward health, an interesting question began to haunt me: *How well am I really following Jesus physically?* How well are you?

If I had been hanging out with Jesus during his time on earth, I wouldn't have been able to keep up with him. He was a fit guy. He walked everywhere, never shying away from the long journeys. One New Testament researcher added together all of the miles that Jesus is documented as having walked and estimates that he averaged at least twenty miles per day during his three years of active ministry.[1] I would have been left gasping in his sandal dust.

In the process of getting myself fit, I had to come to a place where I was ready to follow after Jesus physically. I had to give him this major area I had been withholding. But like the verse says, this meant *turning from my selfish ways*, which wasn't easy. I was too much like the people Paul mentions in his letter to the Philippians:

They are headed for destruction. Their god is their appetite...
—Philippians 3:19

My appetite had certainly become my god. And I was headed for destruction. If I had continued to overeat and never exercise, I was going to die an early death. Now, of course, God is sovereign and ultimately in control of our time on earth, but I had become one of the many people who use his sovereignty as a big, fat excuse to trash my body. God also says that we will reap what we sow.

If you and I ignore what the Bible says about how to treat our bodies—if we poison them with junk and let them atrophy from lack of use—we put ourselves at very real risk of having them fail sooner than God may have liked. He gives us that freedom. It's like playing a game of Russian roulette with a loaded gun; eventually, a round is going to go off. At some point, had I not changed my habits, I would have dropped dead of a heart attack or a stroke. Unhealthy habits lead to an early grave. There's no way around it.

On the other hand, Jesus promised that whoever is willing to lose his life for the sake of the cross will save his life. During the hardest parts of my journey, I clung to the fact that if I lived according to how Jesus wanted me to live, I would find my way back to the life he wanted me to have. I knew I had to lose to live. You and I cannot have an abundant life personally or in the ministry while holding on to our grab bag of bad health habits. We have to loosen our grip on that old way of life in order to find a better one.

Commandment Two—Walk in the Spirit

*So I say, let the Holy Spirit guide your lives. Then you won't be
doing what your sinful nature craves.*
—Galatians 5:16

I like to think of walking in the spirit as giving God complete control of my life. My goal is to make the Holy Spirit not just a resident in me but the president of me. I have always been mindful of the spirit's role when I'm preaching, teaching or counseling, but for decades I completely neglected him in areas that didn't have to do with my ministry. For example, I would get up at the crack of dawn on Sunday mornings to prepare myself to preach; to pray for the filling of the Holy Spirit and for God to use me—and he would! Most Sundays, I would feel his presence in a very real way.

But by 12:30 or so, the services were over and it was time to eat. At that point, I assumed the Holy Spirit needed to move to the Midwest and help the pastors getting ready to preach there. I never imagined he would want to join me for lunch. In truth, I needed him as much when I sat down to eat on Sunday afternoons (and during every other meal throughout the week) as I did while preparing for worship on Sunday mornings. I just didn't realize it.

Personally, my sin bent isn't to crave pornography, tobacco, alcohol or gambling. I'm not pulled in by shopping or given to much coveting. The lust of the flesh in my case is a weakness to overeat and to under exercise. I have had to train myself to walk in the spirit every time I walk into a restaurant, a grocery store or even my kitchen. When I acknowledge the Holy Spirit in those places, he is there, ready to help me.

Have you ever prayed while standing in aisle seven? I have. Have you ever prayed while looking at a lunch menu, knowing that your food decisions are ultimately spiritual decisions? Have you ever prayed that what you have for dinner with your family will be honoring to God?

Let me challenge you to start praying for the Holy Spirit to help you choose the right foods rather than praying that he would use the poor choices on your plate to nourish you despite their lack of nutritional value. That seems a little backwards anyway, doesn't it? There's something off about praying that God would use a pile of deep-fried grease or pseudo-food loaded with sugar to nourish your body; he does generally work within the natural laws he created for us. Thankfully, as Paul promises, when the Holy Spirit is guiding you, you won't give in to what the sinful nature craves.

Commandment Three—Control Your Environment

But put on the Lord Jesus Christ, and make
no provision for the flesh, to fulfill its lusts.
—Romans 13:14 (NKJV)

Commandment Three goes hand-in-hand with Commandment Two. Being intentional about controlling your environment helps keep you in step with the Holy Spirit's guidance in your life. You are setting yourself up for failure if you pray that the spirit would lead you into right food choices, but your cabinets are filled with Oreos and Doritos. No matter how strong your discipline, at some point you are going to have a particularly stressful day and those suckers are going to convince you that they are the perfect remedy for what ails you. But if they aren't there, you can't eat them.

There's one thing I know about myself: *if food gets near me, it will get in me.* Because of that fact, I had to learn to take responsibility for what I allowed into my kitchen. I had to take responsibility for the restaurants I chose to walk into for lunch. And so do you. Whether you do the shopping or your spouse does the shopping, make sure you have agreed on what goes into the grocery cart before you set foot in the store. If certain restaurants tempt you to eat the wrong things, find somewhere new to go. The best way to control your environment is to begin putting simple barriers in place that will help you stick to the health commitments you are making.

Commandment Four—Control Your Portions

If you are a big eater, put a knife to your throat.
—Proverbs 23:2

We suffer from portion distortion in this country. Our portions are out of control. Most restaurant entrées can easily feed two or three people. We know we're eating too much as we wipe the last bit off of our plates, but we do it anyway. Soon, overeating feels like just eating. One of my close friends and former staff members loves to tell the story of when he and another member of my staff were attending a conference with me. We took a break for food at a local fast food burger joint. I stepped up to the counter and ordered three double cheeseburgers, fries and an extra-large drink. Since I ordered three burgers, my two companions thought that I was ordering for them, as well. When I turned around and said, "Your turn to order," they both just stared at me in amazement.

I used to skim past Proverbs 23:2. I avoided it for three reasons. First of all, it's a weird verse (let's face it). Secondly, I was a big eater (obviously). Thirdly, I didn't really like the mental image of a knife to my throat (who would?). One day, I realized I had to take this verse seriously. I'm still not sure I grasp the full implication of it, but there's no doubt that it means to stop eating so much. God is telling us, through his Word, to pay attention to portion control. We should probably listen.

Not too long ago, I visited an exhibition featuring the human body. While I was there, I saw an actual stomach. I was blown away by how small it was. The stomach is the size of a human fist, not the size of a human head. As I sat down to eat that night and looked at the amount of food on my plate, I remembered the stomach I had seen. The memory solidified in my mind the necessity of controlling my portions. Portion control is one of the simplest yet most important steps you and I can take toward health.

Commandment Five—Lay Aside the Weight

Therefore we also, since we are surrounded by so
great a cloud of witnesses, let us lay aside every weight,
and the sin which so easily ensnares us, and let us run with
endurance the race that is set before us.
—Hebrews 12:1 (NKJV)

This verse has often been the springboard for my first-of-the-year messages. I would challenge my congregation to lay aside the weight of bitterness, anger, debt, and the like. I encouraged them to shed those besetting sins so they could run full force toward the abundant life Jesus offers them. It never occurred to me that, along with me, most of them were as hindered as much by physical weight as by anything else.

In this verse, the author of Hebrews mentions that a great cloud of witnesses surrounds us. The saints who have gone before us are watching us to see how we handle life here on earth. Not to mention, our friends are watching us; our church members are watching us; even people who are opposed to God's ways are watching us, hoping they can point a finger and label us as hypocrites.

I'm reminded of Paul's admonition for us to live a life worthy of the calling we have received (Ephesians 4:1). When a body struggling from the consequences of poor health choices ensnares you, you can't live a life worthy of your calling; you can't run the race with endurance. What you eat or fail to eat, how much you exercise or fail to exercise, how much you rest or don't rest, how well you handle stress or don't handle it—all of these things may happen in private, but their effects are evident to the on-looking world. We bring the weight on ourselves, but we can also lay it aside if we will choose to. Because we are surrounded, we have a responsibility to live well—not only for our own sakes, but also for all of those who are looking to our example.

Commandment Six—Control Your Thoughts

*We destroy every proud obstacle that keeps people
from knowing God. We capture their rebellious
thoughts and teach them to obey Christ.*
—2 Corinthians 10:5

What you eat starts in your mind. You know how it is: a certain food pops into your head and suddenly you start craving it. You can't stop thinking about how good it sounds. Before long, you've decided that's what you are going to have for lunch or dinner. In short order, a seed that was planted in your mind turns into an oversized portion on your plate.

Believe me, I've been there. When it came to reigning in my unhealthy habits, I had to learn how to bring every thought into captivity—not only thoughts about food, but also negative thoughts about exercise, excuses about not sleeping and worry over the problems I was facing. I had to come to terms with the fact that, even if three cheeseburgers were swirling around in my mind, that didn't mean they needed to become a reality in my stomach. I could redirect my thoughts to something more beneficial and then act on those more beneficial thoughts. So can you.

Short-term pleasure is not worth long-term pain.

Changing the way you think is key to changing your life for the better. Fill your mind with information and knowledge about healthy living. Reading something about health and wellness every day is a great way to keep your focus right and help you stay on track. Make an intentional effort to block out those late nights commercials for pizza and burgers and instead fill your mind with mantras that will continually remind you of your goal. Here's one I have repeated to myself countless times: *Short-term pleasure is not worth long-term pain.* This one thought has helped me make right choices more than any other thought. Maybe it will help you do the same.

Also, don't forget to read and meditate on God's Word. Take the scriptures from these Ten Commandments and commit them to memory. If you will seal them in your heart and think on them often, God will help you keep your thought life pure and honoring to him.

Commandment Seven—Glorify God

*So whether you eat or drink, or whatever you do,
do it all for the glory of God.*
—1 Corinthians 10:31

This verse is a great litmus test for every decision you make about what to consume. When you pull something off of the supermarket shelf, ask yourself, "Does this choice bring glory to God?" When you sit down at your favorite dive and decide what to order, ask it again. Intimidating, huh? Once I started asking myself this question, I had to put things back on the shelf more than once. I had to call the waiter back over and change my order a few times, too.

If you aren't careful, food can quickly set itself up as an idol. But when you start thinking about how God feels about the food choices you're making—about which of your choices bring him honor and glory and which don't—your perspective changes; your mind snaps back to the fact that your body isn't your own. Every bite you put in your mouth has consequences that will ultimately honor or dishonor the body God created and gave you to manage. In every choice you make, in every bite you take, glorify him.

Commandment Eight—Be a Vessel for Honor

*If you keep yourself pure, you will be a special utensil for
honorable use. Your life will be clean, and you will be ready
for the Master to use you for every good work.*
—2 Timothy 2:21

God has prepared you for many good works in the future but, to accomplish those good works, you have to have a future. Makes sense, doesn't it? Some of us are never going to fulfill the good work that God has for us because we do not honor him with our bodies;

we do not keep our vessels pure in order to be his tools for honorable use. That's on us. Decisions on our part determine whether we are qualified and ready to do what he wants us to do. God has an abundance of work ready and waiting for you. The question is, can you get it all done in the shape you're in?

God has blessed you with one body, one vessel, one life to live for him. When that body has all it can take, you don't get a do-over—not on this earth anyway. You only have one heart, are you taking care of it? You only have one brain, are you protecting and utilizing it? You only have one digestive tract, are you overloading it? If you die as a result of negligent living, you won't be able to take care of the flock God has entrusted to you; you won't be around for your family; you won't be able to influence your world in all the ways God had in store. You have a choice in the matter. You play a major role. Choose to do your part to be prepared for the good work he has planned for you.

Commandment Nine—Run and Walk

But those who trust in the lord will find new strength.
They will soar high on wings like eagles. They will run
and not grow weary. They will walk and not faint.
—Isaiah 40:31

When I went back to the gym for the first time after years of not exercising, it was a humbling experience. I got on the treadmill and all I could do was five minutes. That was it. I thought I was going to pass out. Here I was, someone who used to run for hours at practice, and now I was hyperventilating after only a few minutes of low-level exertion. (More on that story later.) I had to trust God to renew my strength and to give me both the motivation and the sheer physical stamina I needed to get back in shape. I knew that without his help, running—even walking—would never be easy for me again.

As motivation to start getting my strength back, I set an early goal to finish a 5K (3.1 miles) run/walk. This was a big deal for someone who could only do five minutes on a treadmill. I didn't just look for a 5K to participate in; I decided to create my own "Losing to Live 5K" in my town. How's that for a kick in the backside? If you are the guy putting on the 5K, you had better be able to complete it with a little dignity.

I'm happy to say that, after a lot of perseverance and quite a struggle to start walking and then running again, I did it. I finished my first "Losing to Live 5K." (Now the event is an annual hoorah with thousands of participants.) God truly renewed my strength. As I crossed that finish line, having trusted in his grace to sustain me as I did what it took to reach my goal, I felt like I was flying high on wings like eagles.

Commandment Ten—Present Your Body to God

And so, dear brothers and sisters, I plead with you to give your bodies to God because of all he has done for you. Let them be a living and holy sacrifice—the kind he will find acceptable. This is truly the way to worship him.
—Romans 12:1

This commandment speaks to the imperative you and I have to surrender our bodies to God (see Chapter 3). Throughout the Bible, God provides many examples of how we can use our specific body parts to honor him. He mentions how our feet, hands, mouths, eyes, minds, and hearts can bring him glory. But in order for that to happen, we have to give all of those body parts back to the one who created them.

Before you can effectively present your body to God, you have to make sure you have truly surrendered every bit of it to him, as we've discussed. Are you allowing your body to be a holy and living sacrifice? Have your feet taken you anywhere you shouldn't be going? Have your eyes been looking at anything they shouldn't be seeing? Have you given your heart to someone or something that you shouldn't? Have you been putting food in your mouth that harms your temple? You get the idea. Spend some time with God and ask him to help you do a bit of hard self-examination. Tell him you want to be a living and holy sacrifice and ask him to help you get there. Then, let him take control of your body—lifestyle habits and all. (For a handy one-page print-out of the *Ten Commandments for Healthy Living*, go to HealthyRenegade.com.)

Small Steps to Life

- Memorize and meditate on the *Ten Commandments for Healthy Living* scripture verses.

- Pray for the filling of the Holy Spirit when making food choices at the grocery store or when eating out.

- Spend 5 minutes a day reading something on health and wellness

- Memorize this mantra: Short-term pleasure is not worth long-term pain.

· · ·

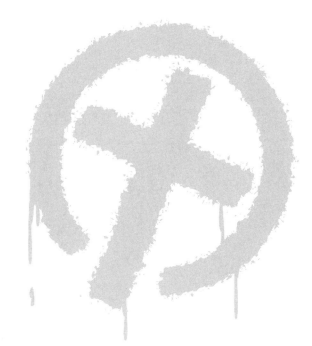

Eating for Life

7

Eating for Life:
Exposing the Acceptable Sin

The religious lifestyle has long been considered a healthy one,
with its constraints on sexual promiscuity, alcohol and tobacco use. . . .
However, overeating may be one sin that pastors and priests regularly overlook.
KENNETH FERRARO (PURDUE SOCIOLOGY PROFESSOR)

Sodom's sins were pride, gluttony, and laziness, while the poor
and needy suffered outside her door. She was proud and committed
detestable sins, so I wiped her out, as you have seen.
EZEKIEL 16:49-50

There's an unaddressed sin undermining church leaders today—
one we've come to accept as normal, even though it has the potential to completely derail the work God has called us to. It's not
what you would expect; not an addiction to drugs, alcohol or
Internet porn, even though those struggles are very real for some.
No, this issue is sneakier. It cloaks itself in a shroud of normalcy
and engages us in a daily battle so subtle that many of us don't
even realize we're at war.

This sin tiptoes into our days in the form of cakes and cookies
brought to the office by well-meaning church members, large glasses
of sweet tea sweating on our desks on hot summer days, the potluck
table filled with creamy casseroles and fried fixings. It thrives thanks
to our almost universal addiction to sugar, to fat and to refined

carbohydrates—to all of those things that excite our taste buds, course into our bodies, make us feel good for a moment and then leave us a little thicker around the middle, a little unhealthier than before, a little less vibrant and less ready to tackle the work God has placed before us.

Have you guessed it yet? The sin is gluttony, plain and simple. So prevalent that it has become a cultural norm, gluttony can be easily overlooked and accepted as a normal part of life. You may not think you have a sin relationship with food and, sure, yours may not be as severe as the next guy's, but if you are a church leader in America, the odds are not in your favor.

Remember the weight statistics from chapter 1? Close to 80% of us are overweight or obese. That's a staggering percentage—and it's simply not acceptable for a group of people who are supposed to be shining the light of God's excellence to an on-looking world. We are called to a higher standard. How have we let ourselves slip so far from where we should be?

Picking and Choosing

The American church is notorious for picking the sins we want to make a big deal out of and overlooking the ones that don't bother us so much. Gluttony is a classic case of that type of thinking. While it is just as much a sin as theft or pride or drunkenness, we have chosen to give it a wink and a smile as we pass through the buffet line over-filling our plates. Can you imagine if 80% of America's pastors were involved in money laundering or illicit affairs? It's unthinkable. The church would collapse. We would be called hypocrites and run out of town. Biblically and culturally, we—along with most Americans—understand just how unacceptable those sins are.

Yet, while gluttony is also unacceptable biblically, it has become an accepted vice culturally. Not only do we embrace this sin, we like to get together and commit it. While we stand and preach against other sins that harm our bodies, we don't have any problem stuffing ourselves to excess each and every day and then parading our bulging bellies—the public evidence of our downfall—around for all to see. Some would say that we are testing God with our stubborn, gluttonous ways. In fact, scripture says it:

> *They stubbornly tested God in their hearts,*
> *demanding the foods they craved.*
> —Psalm 78:18

Sure, we have a hundred excuses (see chapter 4) as to why our weight and health problems aren't our fault. We look to the ways and wisdom of the world to justify our eating choices, following the course the world sets for us every step of the way. Every weekend, many of us promise ourselves that we'll start eating better on Monday. But when Monday rolls around, nothing has changed so nothing changes. We fall into the same pattern we are used to—a pattern of eating what we want, when we want, to the point of excess. And Satan smiles.

Defending Our Sin

Some skilled biblical debaters among us use the Bible to try to argue their way around taking care of their bodies. They claim that, based on scripture, we have permission to eat whatever we'd like. They point to one passage in particular:

> *'It's not what goes into your body that defiles you;*
> *you are defiled by what comes from your heart.'*
> *Then Jesus went into a house to get away from the crowd,*
> *and his disciples asked him what he meant by the parable*
> *he had just used. 'Don't you understand either?'*
> *he asked. 'Can't you see that the food you put into your*
> *body cannot defile you? Food doesn't go into your heart, but*
> *only passes through the stomach and then goes into*

> *the sewer.' (By saying this, he declared that every kind of*
> *food is acceptable in God's eyes.)*
> —Mark 7:15-19

A close examination of this passage shows that the overt leniency argument is not the right interpretation. As you know, the Old Testament is filled with specific dietary laws concerning what is acceptable to eat and what isn't. Most of these laws focus on clean versus unclean meats. Later in scripture, the book of Acts records a vision God gave to Peter, in which he told Peter that all meats had been declared clean (Acts 10:9-16). Mark's account above alludes to that declaration. Jesus is underscoring the point God was making with the vision to Peter: a person can't be defiled by what goes into his stomach—spiritually speaking, that is.

Countless Christians point to this passage, and to Peter's vision, to prove that they have permission to eat whatever and however they would like. "Food can't defile me," they say. "God said I could eat anything I want, so pass me a fork." Unfortunately, this argument is based on a complete misinterpretation of scripture. The vision God gave to Peter, and Jesus' reference to it in Mark, are both making the point that we are no longer spiritually bound by dietary laws.

> Paying attention to what God says about food gives us the greatest chance for optimal health.

The verses are referring specifically to holiness in the eyes of God. By declaring all things clean, God mandated that there are no longer direct spiritual implications for eating something that was once considered off-limits. Thanks to that mandate, dietary restrictions no longer make or keep us holy. But that doesn't mean that the wisdom contained within them can't help keep us healthy.

What's interesting is that most of the Old Testament laws concerning food coincide with what modern science tells us about the healthiest ways to eat. And why wouldn't they? God designed our bodies, designed food for them and then put his dietary guidelines in place for our own good. Anatomically speaking, paying attention to what he says about food gives us the greatest chance for optimal health. For example:

- Eat lots of fruits and vegetables. (Genesis 1:29)

- Fish with scales and fins are healthier than sea scavengers. (Lev. 11:9-11)

- Pigs don't digest the toxins they eat, so their meat isn't healthy. (Lev. 11:7-8)

- Eat wholesome, life-giving breads. (Ezekiel 4:9)

And the list goes on. As Dr. Rex Russell wrote in *What the Bible Says About Healthy Living*:

> *The primary message of both the Old and the New Testaments is salvation; and salvation comes through the blood sacrifice of the Messiah, not through eating habits. Nevertheless, a large portion of the Scripture focuses on commands, ordinances and statutes that show us how to live on this carefully designed earth. Many of these passages pertain to subjects such as economics, law, government, interpersonal relationships, nutrition and health. The sacrifice Jesus made for our sins does not cancel the wisdom in these other teachings. As Paul said, they are still profitable.*[1]

To be sure, the foods you and I choose to eat no longer influence our spiritual standing in God's eyes, but that reality has nothing to do with how those foods—and the sheer quantity of them that we consume—affect our physical health and wellbeing. As Paul wrote:

You say, 'I am allowed to do anything'—but not everything is good for you. And even though 'I am allowed to do anything,' I must not become a slave to anything.
—1 Corinthians 6:12

Have you become a slave to what you put in your mouth? It's easy to do—and it's even easier to justify in today's food culture. But God has a better plan. He has a plan to use the foods he created for you to your benefit; to allow you to walk in health and vibrancy as you honor him with how you treat your body.

Be careful of letting others convince you that God isn't concerned with the dietary choices you make. When it comes to your health, those choices are vitally important—and your health, as we've seen, is one of the greatest tools in God's arsenal for doing his work on this earth.

Making excuses and using scripture to smokescreen the sin you and I love leaves us playing right into our enemy's hands. There's nothing he would rather do than convince us that God is okay with us overloading our bodies with the foods that will eventually kill us. After all, when our bodies fail, then we are out of service. As healthy renegades, let's decide to stop making excuses for our pervasive gluttony and get on with living a better life for the glory of God.

Small Steps to Life
• Repent of the gluttonous habits in your life.
• Acknowledge that God's understanding of your physical health needs surpasses your own.
• Decide to stop justifying unhealthy lifestyle choices.

• • •

Healthy Renegade Pastor Profile

Jimmy Britt
Rocky River Church, Concord, NC

I am forty-six years old and have been in full-time ministry for twenty-two years. I have struggled with my weight all of my life. I finally got to the point where all of my numbers, blood pressure and sugar in particular, were going the wrong way. I was on blood pressure medications, had sleep apnea and my body was preparing for diabetes. I finally realized that I needed help or I was going to die. I was a heart attack or a stroke waiting to happen. I weighed 384 pounds, and I knew I had to do something.

My biggest struggle is mental. I still struggle with wanting to eat until my mind, not just my stomach, is full. I also struggle with making my health a priority, even though I know it needs to be high on the list. Being in ministry makes weight management and healthy living harder. Here are a few reasons why:

1. We have a church culture that celebrates (unhealthy) food. It seems like every event and church meeting centers around food.

2. *Pulpit bumpers* (aka big bellies) are accepted by our church folks. There do not seem to be the same health stigmas for pastors that exist in other executive professions.

3. Pastors and churchgoers don't know what the Bible says about health, so there is no spiritual connection between overeating and your relationship with Jesus. You and I know what the Bible says about the sins we take seriously, like alcohol abuse and pornography, but when was the last time you heard a sermon on gluttony?

Thankfully, I have been able to lose almost 150 pounds and currently weigh 235. However, I still have my struggles to deal with. I am still working on better discipline and ongoing mentor accountability. I have to keep working at having an ongoing plan and strategy for staying healthy.

It is important for Christians to understand that poor physical health hampers what we can do in ministry just like poor financial health. For example, God could not call many of us to the mission field because we could not afford to go. We are too far in debt. Likewise, many people disqualify themselves from ministry simply because they do not have the personal stamina to be able to handle it.

I have learned that if you are unhealthy and overweight, you are putting limits on what God can and will do in your life. Get help, especially if you are obese, morbidly obese, or super morbidly obese. Find a doctor who cares about your life, if you do not have one already. Get the data on where your health is.

I recently challenged the people at Rocky River Church to go to the next level in their relationship with God. This challenge was a commitment to weekly worship, to reading all four gospels, to participating in a Growth Group, to tithing and some other important things necessary to grow spiritually. As a part of this challenge, I asked our church to make a commitment to work on their physical health as well. Amazing things happened. We had men and women losing weight all over our church. In fact, because it was so impactful, we plan to kick off next year with a healthy living message series, Growth Groups, and weekly weigh-ins that will be church and community wide. I cannot wait to report on the tonnage of fat that will melt away.

Jimmy's Advice: Take your health seriously. Don't let it run out before God is finished with you.

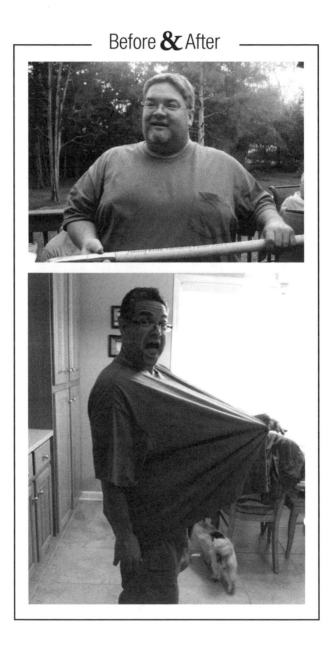

8

Eating for Life:
How Renegades Eat

You have a clear choice. You can live longer and healthier than
ever before, or you can do what most modern populations do;
eat to create disease and a premature death.
DR. JOEL FUHRMAN (AUTHOR, EAT TO LIVE)

So whether you eat or drink, or whatever you do,
do it all for the glory of God.
—1 CORINTHIANS 10:31

The birth of a child always seems to bring new perspective. If you
have children, think about the moments after they popped into the
world. While you likely believed in the miracle of God's divine creation before the birth, something about seeing a new life emerge
before your eyes wakes you up to just how incredible God is—and
just how much care he has put into creating the intricacies that make
up each one of us. Pause for a moment and really consider the mag-
nitude of King David's words about our formation:

> *For You formed my inward parts; You covered*
> *me in my mother's womb. I will praise You,*
> *for I am fearfully and wonderfully made.*
> —Psalm 139:13-14 (NKJV)

You and I are products of a generous, intelligent Creator who fashioned each one of us in his image. He gave us breath and then offered us a world that he created specifically to sustain us in health and wholeness. He gave us food for nourishment and water to quench our thirst. He told us to get busy working the land. Thanks to these gifts, our ancestors—those who ate a more primitive diet and engaged in a more active lifestyle than we do—often lived to a vibrant, healthy old age.

The picture is very different today. As a society, we are making collective daily health choices that, over the last few decades, have put us on a downward spiral toward chronic illness and early death. A hundred years ago, lifestyle-related diseases such as diabetes, heart disease and even cancer were practically unheard of. In many cultures—those that have never stopped eating the way generations before us did—that's still the case. Yet, for those of us living in modern westernized countries, these types of diseases have become commonplace.

> Most of the ailments filling our prayer request lists are reversible—better yet, altogether preventable—with some simple dietary changes.

Like fish in water, most of us have a hard time seeing the nature of the environment we live in. If only we could grasp the truth that we are bringing the pain of poor health on ourselves; that most of the ailments filling our prayer request lists are reversible (better yet, altogether preventable) with some simple dietary changes. We are what we eat—literally. And what we eat is killing us at an astounding rate. It's time to get back to the basics and begin nourishing our bodies the way God intended.

Back to Basics

What if you woke up tomorrow morning to find the car of your dreams sitting in your driveway? Imagine that an anonymous do-gooder heard you'd always wanted a Porsche (or a Lamborghini, or a top-of-the-line Ford F-150… whatever it may be) and decided to thank you for all of your hard work by leaving one parked where your old car sat the night before. How excited would you be?

I bet you would treat that car like a prized possession. You would keep it clean; you wouldn't let the kids eat in it; you would make sure the oil was changed regularly and that all of the fluid levels were in check; and you would give it the fuel that the manufacturer meant for it to have, wouldn't you? There's no way you would risk harming that machine by filling it with lower grade fuel than it needed to function like it's supposed to. After all, not only would that be a slap in the face to the person who gave you the gift, but it would also keep you from enjoying your new toy at peak performance for as long as possible.

Amazingly, you and I—along with most Americans—fully grasp this concept when it comes to taking care of an automobile, but when it comes to our own bodies we conveniently fail to make the connection. Here's the reality: When you woke up this morning, God gave you a great gift. He gave you an intricately designed body specifically crafted for the purpose of being his representative on this earth. He gave you breath to fill your lungs and a pumping heart to circulate your blood. He gave you a mind capable of more than you can fathom. He placed your soul (and his spirit!) in this meticulously crafted machine and handed it over to you as a gift. How are you treating it? Are you treating it as well as you would treat that car? What kind of fuel are you putting in it on a daily basis to make sure it operates at peak performance for the long haul?

When you eat the foods that fuel your body well, you are cooperating with God to be a good steward of the vessel he has entrusted to you. Unfortunately, cultural persuasion and free will have thwarted

God's best intentions for the majority of us—but it's not too late. We can get back to the health God desires us to have. We can work with him rather than against him by making better choices, starting today. Barring miracles, God won't do this for us. To do so, he would have to go against the natural laws of cause and effect that he put in place. But, if you and I will do our part to be healthy, we can trust him to bless our efforts.

Part of the problem is that we overcomplicate the issue. God's prescription for health is really pretty simple: Eat the foods he created in the closest possible form to their original creation. In other words, eat an apple, not an apple fritter. Eat a piece of wild salmon, not a microwavable fish stick. As Jordan Rubin wrote in *The Maker's Diet*:

> *Most Americans eat great quantities of food frequently, based on convenience. In fact, the entire fast food and TV dinner industries have flourished due to our fast-paced lifestyles.... Unfortunately, the Creator didn't design our bodies to operate at optimum levels on junk food, fast food, or prepackaged foods. His laws that govern our entire human nature, including our health, bring consequences when violated, whether or not we accept the fact that they are still in place.*[1]

To reclaim our health and begin functioning the way God intended, we have to get back to his original plan for our eating habits. We have to get back to basics. Here are three overarching guidelines that, if incorporated into our thinking on a daily basis, can revolutionize our health and put us back on the track to physical wellbeing:

1. Eat Living Foods

Then God said, 'Look! I have given you every seed-bearing plant throughout the earth and all the fruit trees for your food.'
—Genesis 1:29

Living foods are the life-giving fruits, vegetables, beans and grains God created specifically to fuel our bodies. They contain nutrients and enzymes designed to work within our anatomical systems to sustain health and energy. In their natural state, fruits, vegetables, beans and grains are so nutritionally complex that many of the healthful compounds within them haven't even been identified. For example, a tomato contains more than ten thousand different phyto-chemicals, all of which work together to benefit the body.[2] The range and composition of these phyto-chemicals is so complex that scientists are still trying to identify the details of God's craftsmanship.

Processed, packaged foods, on the other hand can be characterized as dead foods. While living foods are foods that God made, dead foods are foods produced or drastically altered (think potato chips rather than fresh potatoes) by humans. The name is apropos because not only do they contain no living energy, but if you eat enough of them you will find yourself on the fast track toward sickness and death. Just think about it: If something can sit on a supermarket shelf for months (oftentimes years) and still be considered "safe" to eat, there is obviously no life in it. Living things die. That food is nothing but a combination of chemicals and preservatives wrapped up in an appealing package and laced with sugar and salt to keep you and me going back for more.

> Good health doesn't happen by chance; it is earned one bite at a time.

The first key to reclaiming or maintaining optimal health is to fill your plate with living foods. Eat fruits and vegetables. Eat beans and whole grains. Make sure your food choices include a lot of color—or, as it is sometimes said, *eat a rainbow everyday*. Green, red, orange, and yellow fruits and vegetables will fill you with living energy and flood your system with the building blocks of superior health. When your diet includes large quantities of the living foods God made, you are not only staving off obesity and all of its negative outcomes, you are also proactively fortifying your cells against disease—particularly against cancer.

In many scientific circles, cancer has come to be known as a "Fruit and Vegetable Deficiency Disease." The *Journal of the National Cancer Institute* recently reported that men who ate three or more servings of cruciferous vegetables per week, such as broccoli and cabbage, had a 41% reduced risk of prostate cancer compared with those who ate less than one serving.[3] That's a significant reduction! When the same men added a variety of other vegetation to their diets, the risk went down even more.

If someone created a pill that slashed cancer risk by close to 50%, everyone in America would want to take it. Yet, we can accomplish the same thing through being wise about what we put in our mouths and we just don't do it. Why? Taste? Culture? Inertia? These are all weak excuses for failing to cooperate with God to maintain our health.

Speaking of pills: Many people think that if they take a multivitamin, they don't need to eat their fruits and vegetables. While vitamins are an important part of a healthy lifestyle, no vitamin can duplicate the unique nutrient composition found in whole fruits and vegetables—a combination of synergistic elements (antioxidants, flavonoids, phytonutrients, etc.) that work in the body to minimize inflammation, destroy harmful cells and bolster health. Focus your energy on nutrient-rich foods, not isolated, scientifically extracted "nutrients." Good health doesn't come in a bottle or happen by chance; it is earned one bite at a time.

2. Trade White for Whole Grain

*Now go and get some wheat, barley, beans, lentils, millet,
and emmer wheat, and mix them together in a storage jar.
Use them to make bread for yourself…*
—Ezekiel 4:9

You may have heard the expression, "If it's white, don't bite." This quirky phrase came about with good reason. Refined carbohydrates, such as white bread, white rice, white pastas and most baked goods are one of the major culprits behind America's weight and sickness epidemic.

Not all carbohydrates are created equal. The carbohydrates found in fruits, vegetables, beans and whole grains are known as complex carbohydrates and are essential building blocks of health. But the refined (read: processed) carbohydrates so prevalent today are dangerous beyond measure. They have had all of the nutritional value stripped out of them. What remains is nothing but sugar—literally. When refined carbohydrates enter your body, they are converted directly to sugar, which is why they are responsible for so many obesity-related diseases.

Consider this study: Over a period of six years, scientists tracked 43,000 men whose diets were high in white rice, white bread and white pasta. The participants had two and a half times the incidence of Type II diabetes as those who ate high-fiber alternatives such as whole grain bread and brown rice.[4] Type II diabetes is nothing to be taken lightly. It is the seventh leading cause of death in America[5]— and completely preventable. In addition to obesity and diabetes, these nutritionally defunct foods also lead to higher incidences of heart disease and many types of cancer.[6]

As you begin to fill your diet with more living foods, also be intentional about cutting out refined carbohydrates. Opt instead for whole grain products. Whole grain varieties (which are also complex carbohydrates) retain the fiber and nutrients that have been stripped from white carbohydrates, so they interact with your body in an entirely different way. One note of caution: Be wary of breads and other baked goods that are simply labeled "whole wheat." Those are often just white bread products with a little coloring added. Make sure you read the nutrition label, and only buy products where whole grain components are first on the list of ingredients.

3. Limit Animal Protein

Do not mix with winebibbers, Or with gluttonous eaters of
meat; For the drunkard and the glutton will come to poverty...
—Proverbs 23:20-21

Don't worry. I'm not going to tell you that you need to become a vegetarian. But I am going to recommend that you begin practicing some significant moderation when it comes to the amount of meat you eat. To say that the amount of animal protein you and I consume is significantly higher than that of generations past is a huge understatement—and this extreme increase in quantity is directly responsible for many of the health problems we struggle with today.

A hundred years ago, meat was more of a treat than a staple. Sunday dinner was special because it was usually the only meal of the week where meat was served. These days, however, we've come to believe that a meal isn't complete unless it includes meat. As a result, most Americans are eating meat at least twice, if not three times, every single day—and in large quantities, to boot.

This is problematic on a couple of levels. First of all, thanks to the saturated fat that is synonymous with animal protein, the large quantities of meat we eat directly correlate with the skyrocketing rates of heart disease and various cancers we're facing in this country. Second, the more meat we fill up on, the less vegetables and whole grains we are going to eat—so we are trading the nutritional benefits contained in those for something that's not nearly as beneficial to our health. Writing about the findings of *The China Project*, the most comprehensive study ever done on the relationship between diet and disease, Dr. Joel Fuhrman, a leading specialist on disease prevention and reversal, noted:

> *The data showed huge differences in disease rates based on the amount of plant foods eaten and the availability of animal products. Researchers found that as animal foods increased in*

the diet...so did the emergence of the cancers that are common in the West. Most cancers occurred in direct proportion to the quantity of animal foods consumed. ...

All animal products are low (or completely lacking) in the nutrients that protect us against cancer and heart attacks—fiber, antioxidants, phytochemicals, folate, Vitamin E, and plant proteins. They are rich in substances that scientific investigations have shown to be associated with cancer and heart disease incidence: saturated fat, cholesterol, and arachidonic acid.[7]

The amount of cholesterol and saturated fat that most of us consume from animal sources significantly outweighs the amount of healthful nutrients we consume from plant sources. This reality is leading us down paths of sickness and premature death much more quickly than any meat-loving American wants to admit. Dr. Fuhrman added:

Never forget that coronary artery disease and its end result— heart attacks, the number one killer of all American men and women—are almost 100 percent avoidable. ....most of the poorer countries, which invariably consume small amounts of animal products, have less than 5 percent of the adult population dying of heart attacks. ...the major risk factors associated with heart disease—smoking, physical inactivity, eating processed food, and animal-product consumption—are avoidable. Every heart attack death is even more of a tragedy because it likely could have been prevented.[8]

One of the wisest steps you can take in your journey toward improved health and wellness is to cut back on your meat consumption, both red and white. No, you don't have to eliminate meat altogether, but keeping your helping to less than 10% of your diet—and filling that new gap with fresh vegetables, fruits, beans and grains (not pasta and French fries)—will put you squarely on the path to renegade wellness. (For a free resource on how this connects with the biblical concept of fasting, go to HealthyRenegade.com.)

These three tweaks to your diet are simple, but that doesn't necessarily mean they are easy. The way you eat today is the result of years of conditioning. There will be a learning curve while you retrain your taste buds to enjoy flavors you may not have been exposed to very much. You will also likely experience a few withdrawal symptoms as you cut out refined carbohydrates and their sugary counterparts. Right now, your body is literally addicted to those things and the bond has to be broken.

You can do this. The other side of the mountain is worth the journey it takes to get there. Now is the time for you to control your eating habits rather than letting them control you. Now is the time to take a proactive role in reclaiming your health. Now is the time to begin eating like a renegade!

Small Steps to Life

- Add more colorful fruits and vegetables into a few meals this week.

- Start reading nutrition labels on breads, pastas and baked goods. Only buy products that are 100% whole grain.

- Replace white rice with brown rice.

- Try skipping meat at breakfast and lunch, and only having it for dinner.

. . .

Healthy Renegade Pastor Profile

Jeff Newman
Austin Vineyard Church, Austin, TX

I am sixty-four years old and have been in full-time ministry for forty-two years. I have struggled with maintaining a healthy lifestyle and weight for about thirty years. My story is one of the trials and tribulations that a church planter goes through to establish a church. My wife, Sandra, and I started the Austin Vineyard in 1986. Despite the pressures of ministry, we eventually realized our dream for a viable and sustainable work.

While we reaped success in our efforts, we also reaped premature illness as the result of the stress. I had picked up bad habits of overeating and a lack of regular exercise. My problem was never sweets; it was refilling my plate several times. The weight gain did not happen all at once. It was a gradual, fifteen-year process of becoming obese.

In my early forties, I developed a painful condition called gout. I was also in the beginning stages of Type II Diabetes. This jolted me into trying to lose a few pounds and change my diet. It did not last long. I slipped back into my old patterns of unhealthy eating and little exercise.

Diabetes is a silent killer; it affects every organ in your body. Eventually, I developed high blood pressure, high cholesterol, and the beginning of congestive heart failure. I ended up having several heart stress tests, several nuclear stress tests and two coronary angioplasties to open narrow and blocked heart arteries. I was on seven different prescriptions and had a team of doctors working on my health challenges. One of my doctors repeatedly said to me, "Jeff, you need to lose weight!" But I was hopelessly stuck.

About two years ago, a church leader challenged me to see a weight coach that was helping him lose weight. I was reluctant to go, but I could not deny the results my friend was getting. That decision changed my life. I tipped the scales at 290 pounds when I finally made the move to get healthy. To date, I have lost eighty pounds.

Before I started working with a weight coach, I had an exercise trainer that was working with me three days a week. After several months of intense sessions, my trainer informed me that my problem was in the kitchen, and unless I conquered my eating habits, all the exercise in the world was not going to help. Sometimes the long hours of meeting the needs of a growing church resulted in me making unwise food choices. My favorite fast food was Wendy's. I could not get enough of the *Baconator*! I had to change the way I ate. I had to stop eating myself to death in an attempt to ease my ministry hurts and pains.

As a pastor, I am constantly invited into people's homes and out to restaurants by the church family. Also, a lot of church ministry revolves around food. I cannot tell you how many church potlucks I have been a part of. I have to constantly make healthy choices. Just like I plan my day from my ministry calendar, I also plan my day around what I am going to eat. As for exercise, I turn my daily schedule into walking opportunities. My goal is ten thousand steps per day.

I am now committed to teaching my congregation how to overcome these issues. One of the most effective things I have done for them is to practice a healthy lifestyle myself. They see it every week when I step into the pulpit. I also make it a regular routine to teach on stress management throughout the year. I have added weight competitions to my church calendar and have been exposing the congregation to health professionals who share diet and exercise tips. We have also hosted mobile medical examination services for our local community, as well as for our church community.

Overweight pastor, you can do this! You can break the cycle of obesity in your life, but you cannot do it by yourself. If you will find a group of people who are tired of living mediocre lives, that want to live the life Jesus promised, life more abundant, you can make the changes that will impact not only your personal health but the health of many in your congregation!

Jeff's Advice: Decide now to start eating healthy. Remember, you are not invincible!

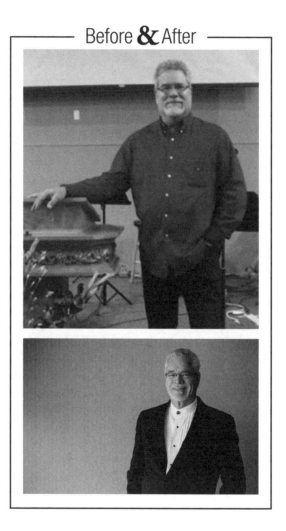

9

Eating for Life:
Avoid Common Pitfalls

We become what we want to be by consistently
being what we want to become each day.
RICHARD G. SCOTT

Forgetting the past and looking forward to what lies ahead,
I press on to reach the end of the race and receive the heavenly prize
for which God, through Christ Jesus, is calling us.
PHILIPPIANS 3:13-14

Circumstances you aren't prepared for can sabotage even the best of intentions. As you begin on this road toward renegade health, remember that you are creating a new lifestyle. This isn't a quick fix. As with every long journey worth taking, there are bound to be a few setbacks. Don't let those discourage you. Progress, not perfection, is the goal.

If you blow your commitment at one meal, don't think of the whole day as shot. Start again with your next meal. The enemy will try to discourage you when you mess up. He'll try to make you think you should quit. When he whispers defeat in your ear, refocus your attention on Jesus—the one who promises you can do all things through him (Philippians 4:13). *All things*, including losing the extra weight, ridding yourself of lifestyle diseases and reclaiming your health for his glory.

That said, there are a few common pitfalls that try to hinder everyone who commits to changing the way they eat for the better. An early awareness of what those are can help you stand strong against them when they threaten to throw you off balance. These are the four that top the list:

1. A sheer sense of resistance
2. A tendency toward emotional eating
3. Lack of family support
4. Eating out

Let's take a look at each one in detail.

Four Common Pitfalls

1. Resistance

Think back to our two pastors—Rob Renegade and Alex Average. Alex didn't intend to end up in the position he's in. He didn't start out in life thinking, "You know, my goal is to get fat, develop a disease or two and become less effective for the kingdom of God." I bet you didn't either. If you can relate to where Alex is now, it's not because you want to be there. But the unrelenting pull of the average, culturally-acceptable unhealthy lifestyle is real and powerful. The resistance you feel toward taking positive initiative is a live, active force.

Stephen Pressfield, author of *Do the Work* and *The War of Art*, has written at length about the nature of the agency he calls Resistance. Take a look at a couple of his observations:

> *Resistance cannot be seen, heard, touched, or smelled. But it can be felt. … The more important a call or action is to our soul's evolution, the more Resistance we will feel toward pursuing it. Resistance's goal is not to wound or disable. Resistance aims to*

kill. Its target is the epicenter of our being: our genius, our soul,
the unique and priceless gift we were put on this earth to give…[1]

Pressfield's words sound a lot like Jesus' description of the devil
himself. As we've already seen:

> *The thief's purpose is to steal, kill and destroy.*
> —John 10:10

The enemy of your soul is also the enemy of the purposes God has
for you on this earth. He wants to kill you. Period. And he's hoping
he can do that by your own hand. He wants to make you think you
can't change your life. He wants to deceive you into believing that a
couple of unhealthy meals won't matter. Careful, because all he's trying to do is keep you traveling the path toward your own destruction.
He's applying subtle, unrelenting pressure to get you to settle for
your current state of being; for health that looks like everyone else's;
for a life that's lacking the abundance Jesus came to give you. But as
James wrote so plainly:

> *Resist the devil, and he will flee from you.*
> —James 4:7

When the enemy tries to temp you back toward your old way of life,
resist. When resistance pulls you toward grabbing an unhealthy meal
out of convenience rather than taking the time to eat something that
will nourish your body, resist. As you get in the habit of opposing
the enemy's schemes, he will turn his attention toward someone else.
(For more on resisting Satan's lies, turn to chapter 13.)

2. Emotional Eating

We're all guilty of using food to make ourselves feel better. The comfort foods we know and love seem to do a great job of helping us calm

down when we are anxious and picking us up when we've had a rough day—or do they? When we look to food to give us an emotional boost, we may get a momentary surge of pleasure from what we eat, but ultimately we end up feeling worse. Not only are our problems still there, but we also feel guilty about gorging. This can lead to a downward spiral of resignation and even more emotional eating.

Emotional eating is an extremely common problem. In fact, a large percentage of people who struggle with over-eating and excess weight are emotional eaters. As pastors, we are particularly prone to this pitfall. You and I have a hard job, with an extremely emotional component. If you are anything like me, you just want to sit down and decompress when you get home at the end of a challenging day (which is most likely every day). A bag of chips, a pint of ice cream, or dinner's leftovers often seem like the perfect couch companion. But when we allow ourselves to eat out of emotional hunger rather than physical hunger, not only are we are adding to our health problems, we're also failing to deal with the stress in our lives productively.

To begin getting emotional eating under control, figure out what your most common triggers are. What situations or feelings make you want to reach for comfort food? Maybe it's when you are under a lot of stress; maybe your trigger is nothing more than boredom, or even pure habit. Whatever it is for you, start taking intentional note of when your eating is driven by something other than hunger.

Then, when you find yourself reaching for food for all the wrong reasons, learn to pause. Tell yourself you are going to wait ten minutes before having that snack. Use those ten minutes to do something that may help you deal with your emotions in a healthier way. Go for a quick walk. Play with your kids. Talk to your spouse about your day. When those ten minutes have passed, your urge to eat will likely have passed, too—and you will have started decompressing in a much healthier way.

3. Lack of Family Support

Healthy lifestyle habits are much easier to adopt when everyone in your household is on board—but that's not always the way it works. You may find yourself being a lone ranger in a house full of people who have no interest in getting healthier. If that's the case, simply keep your focus steadily trained on why you are going renegade and continue pressing toward your goal.

Your success will eventually have a major impact on the people you love. They may want to sit back and watch for a while, but when they begin seeing the changes in your body, your increase in energy, and your overall improved quality of life, they will want those things for themselves. They will begin asking questions. It's not unlike shining your witness to an unbelieving world. Make the people around you so curious about the positive changes in your life that they want to know what you know.

Practically speaking, if your family isn't with you on this, you may need to take some inconvenient steps to stay on track. If your spouse does the grocery shopping, make sure healthy items get onto the list and into the cart. In addition, designate a separate area of the refrigerator for your healthy foods, so you can get right to them without having to rummage through old temptations.

While going it alone in your home won't be easy, commit to carrying the torch. When you don't falter, not only will you be better for it, but your entire family will benefit as well. They will begin their own healthy journeys in their own time.

4. Eating Out

Restaurant meals can be one of the worst enemies of a health-conscious lifestyle—and in our profession, we end up eating in a lot of restaurants. But with a little pre-planning and a handful of strategies for success, eating out can become part of your healthy routine rather than an excuse for slipping back into your old ways.

First of all, if you know you are going to be eating out, be intentional about choosing a restaurant that will have some healthy options. As much as it is up to you, avoid places where you'll have a hard time finding something you'll feel good about on the menu. Also try to avoid your old haunts, where familiar smells and ingrained habits may push you over the edge of temptation. You may be able to go back to those places one day and order with more wisdom, but don't put yourself in that position too soon.

If you are eating with staff or friends who want to go somewhere that would make it hard on you, don't be shy about suggesting an alternative. If they know that you are committed to getting healthy, they will likely be more than willing to go somewhere different.

Once you are in a restaurant, keep these tips for success in mind:

- *Pray*—Before you order, have a quiet conversation with God. Thank him for the changes he's making in your body and for the newfound health in your life. Ask him to help you choose a meal that will honor him.

- *Focus*—Focus your attention on the healthiest options on the menu. Don't even read about the burger and fries. Look for vegetables, hearty salads and grilled dishes. And don't hesitate to ask your server how something is prepared. If you want to make a special request, go for it. Most restaurants are more than happy to accommodate dietary concerns.

- *Order First*—I know, I know; we are supposed to put others first. But when you are on a mission to get healthy and you're sitting in a restaurant with other people, make an exception. When the server is ready, be quick to order before anyone else does. That way, you won't be tempted to change your order when you hear what those around you are having.

- *Eat Less*—Portions in most restaurants are out of control. Even if you order something deliciously healthy, there will probably be enough of it on your plate to feed you and the person next to you. Decide before the food hits the table that you are not going to eat it all. Renegades don't believe in the "clean plate club" when it means eating two or three times more than your body needs.

Progress, Not Perfection

Remember, setbacks are part of the process on this journey toward renewed health. Learning to navigate your world with an entirely new lifestyle will take some time and practice—and that's okay. Take small steps every day. Be aware of the pitfalls along your path. If you mess up, shake it off and start again. Get a little better week by week. And always keep telling yourself, "Progress, not perfection, is the goal."

Small Steps to Life

- Acknowledge the presence of resistance in your life—and resist it!

- Take a ten-minute pause before snacking to make sure you're actually hungry.

- Claim a corner of the refrigerator for your healthy groceries.

- Choose restaurants that will have healthy options for you. You may even want to look at the menu online before you go, so you know what your options will be.

• • •

Healthy Renegade Pastor Profile

Darrell Koop
The Ridge Fellowship, Leander, TX

I am forty-six years old and have been serving in ministry for the past twenty-one years. My struggle with weight goes all the way back to high school. Growing up, my family ate a steady diet of Mexican food, pizza, fried chicken, and chicken fried steak. Junk foods were snacks and we had dessert or sweets regularly. We didn't think much about food other than how great it tasted.

When I was a senior in high school, my only living grandfather had a heart attack and had to have quadruple bypass surgery. The day I visited him in the hospital, he said, "Son, don't end up like me, having your chest sawed open and pried apart. Don't eat so much bacon and gravy and butter like I have. You're young. You can do better." That had a profound impact on me, but the problem was I loved bacon and gravy and butter. I used to put almost a whole stick in my macaroni and cheese! Still, I knew I needed to change.

I did okay cutting back on fats, because the image of my grandfather in that hospital bed was so powerful. Then, during the mid to late nineties, the "fat free craze" hit, making it trendy to cut back on fat. The problem was that those fat-free foods were loaded with added sugar to give them taste, which did not help my cravings for sweets. I had several failed attempts at dieting, with my weight yo-yoing up and down. Whenever the weight came back, so did my guilt and frustration. I felt stuck, like I was doomed to be overweight forever.

It wasn't until the last few years through Nelson and Steve that I even attributed my weight and food addictions to a spiritual problem. That's when I began asking God to help me. For the first time, I prayed to eat for my health, to lose weight and to live better. It had never dawned on me before to ask God to help me in these areas!

Praying and memorizing powerful scriptures about health and wellness have helped me so much.

Being in full-time ministry makes it harder for me to stay healthy because when I am stressed or anxious, I often open the pantry or refrigerator. The pressures of ministry like performance, conflict, deadlines and difficult people cause me to need a release. Food has been the legal, easy and acceptable vice for Christians. However, I came to the realization that my draw to sweets was an addiction to be avoided just as an addiction to alcohol. I wish that I didn't crave them, but I do. I have to be careful that I am not making food my comfort instead of God.

As pastors, we have few role models of physical health and wellness. Taking care of the physical body is not something that we hear about at conferences or in messages. Frankly, it's ignored. However, our cohorts in ministry all seem to struggle in this area, too. I have had to overcome the misguided notion that I need to do all spiritual work at the expense of working on myself physically. I have to be careful and not think, "I can always get in shape one of these days. Let's work on what is pressing." In reality, my physical health is as pressing as anything.

Throughout this journey, I have learned that in order to be consistent with my health and weight, I have to stay connected to Christ. If I don't, I find that I start reverting back to my old ways. I have had to learn that in my weakness, he is strong. If I forget my need for Christ, I find myself stuffing my face with cookies.

I am passionate about Christians getting healthy. Helping people see that health actually improves all areas of life, including marriage and family life has been beneficial for my congregation. As a pastor, some people think that I should talk only about spiritual things—not diet, exercise and health. I now teach that the spiritual and physical are both important, and that you can't have one without the other. I want people to understand that gluttony and laziness do not honor God. We need to move, set goals, and be good stewards, not only of our money and time, but also of our bodies and energy. I now teach that our vision of showing Christ to others includes every aspect of our lives.

Abundant living starts now, not just in heaven. To feel good, have energy, and live a healthy life in Christ is to walk in what he has for us now. Get started. You can do it! And you will inspire and lead others as you take steps to be healthy. May God do amazing things through you as you are obedient in this area.

Darrell's Advice: Take time to plan for and pray about your health. If you neglect your physical health, you, your family and your congregation will suffer.

Before & After

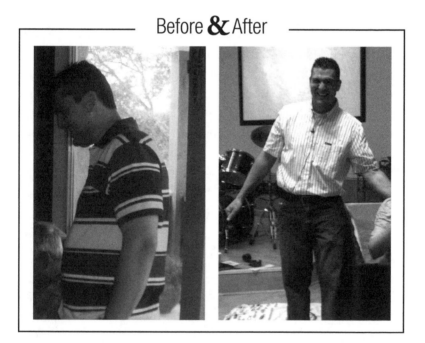

10

Eating for Life:
Drink Up

Pure water is the world's first and foremost medicine.

SLOVAKIAN PROVERB

The earth was formless and empty, and darkness covered the deep waters.
And the Spirit of God was hovering over the surface of the waters.

GENESIS 1:2

When you wake up in the morning and it's pouring rain outside, do you thank God for the deluge or do you think, "Oh no. I have to drive to the office in this!" Most of us lean toward the latter, but really we should be praising God for the incredible gift he's sending us from the sky—the gift of water. Water has been a priority to God from the very beginning. After all, it was the first element on earth (Genesis 1:1-2). But, these days, we underestimate just how important it is to our daily lives and our bodies.

When you consider that our bodies are mostly made of water, it makes sense that water is important for our physical wellbeing. Just think about it: Your brain and heart are 73% water. Your lungs are 83% water. Your skin is 64% water. Your muscles and kidneys are 79% water. Even your bones are 31% water. Because you and I are comprised largely of water, water is necessary for all of our bodily functions. Without enough of it being poured into our systems, our health will, well… dry up.

Dehydration Is Deadly

Three-fourths of Americans walk around chronically dehydrated—so chances are, you are one of them. How often do you feel thirsty? When the feeling of thirst hits you, you are already dehydrated. Dehydration is a dangerous condition. It's the hidden culprit behind many health problems, three of which I (Steve) suffered with greatly when I was at my unhealthiest. You may, too:

Dry Skin—When your body is lacking water, it rations and prioritizes the little bit it does have. The brain and the heart are top priority, so the body makes sure to keep those two things hydrated. But other organs, including your skin (your body's biggest organ), suffer as a result. Despite all of the lotions and creams you and I use to try to keep dry skin at bay, it's an internal problem.

High Blood Pressure—While high blood pressure is mainly a result of poor food choices and other lifestyle issues, dehydration compounds the problem drastically. Blood is 83% water. When you aren't drinking enough, your blood thickens and your heart has to work harder to circulate it. This can compound issues of high blood pressure—as it did in my case—and in some cases even cause high blood pressure in someone who didn't previously have it.

Vocal Chord Damage—When I was at my heaviest weight of 340 pounds, and not drinking water like I should, I damaged my vocal cords. Preaching three services each weekend and failing to stay hydrated led to the development of nodules that I had to have surgically removed. What I did not realize is that water serves as a lubricant, like oil to a car. I was speaking, speaking, speaking but wasn't taking time to properly lubricate the muscles giving me the power to speak. Now, when I am preaching on a Sunday morning, I drink five or six bottles of water over the course of the services in order to keep my vocal cords well oiled. If you are having trouble sustaining your voice through a message or have that dry mouth feeling, I encourage you to adopt the same habit.

The Well of Wellness

When there is enough of it to go around, water accomplishes some amazing things within your body. Water:

- Gives you energy
- Regulates digestion by breaking down and flushing out waste
- Aids weight loss (see below)
- Helps stabilize blood pressure
- Clears toxins from your body
- Reduces the chance of kidney stones
- Helps maintain your body's proper acid and alkaline balance
- Improves focus and metal acuity
- Hydrates your skin and slows down the appearance of aging

This is a pretty impressive list, isn't it? Sometimes, I hear the objection, "I don't like water." Do you like being tired? Do you like having digestive problems? Do you like being constipated? Do you like high blood pressure? Do you like having your acid/alkaline imbalanced? Do you like being overweight? Do you like having dried up, wrinkled skin? Do you like having problems with your kidneys and urinary tract? No? Time to drink some water!

Water and Weight Loss

Any healthy lifestyle plan is going to be focused on diet and exercise, but it must also include a heavy emphasis on drinking substantial amounts of water. Consider these facts about water and weight loss[1]:

- Initial weight loss is largely water loss. You need to drink plenty of water in order to avoid dehydration as those pounds drop away.

- Efficient calorie burning requires an adequate supply of water. Dehydration slows down the fat-burning process.

- Burning calories creates toxins that must be flushed out. Water is essential to getting rid of the toxic build-up that your body needs to eliminate.

- Dehydration causes a reduction in blood volume. A reduction in blood volume causes a reduction in the supply of oxygen to your muscles, which in turn makes you feel tired. You don't want to eat right and exercise when you're tired.

- Water helps maintain muscle tone and lubricates your joints. Proper hydration can help reduce muscle and joint soreness when you start becoming active.

- A healthy diet includes a lot of fiber. Without adequate fluids, this necessary fiber can cause constipation.

- Drinking water with a meal helps you feel full and satisfied more quickly. If you are properly hydrated, you'll be more likely to eat only as much food as your body needs.

Since getting your weight under control is a major first step in being a healthy renegade pastor, you literally can't afford to push water aside. It's essential to your new, healthy lifestyle. Once you get used to drinking it in large quantities, you'll be glad you did. You'll feel cleaner, clearer, and more alert. Your body will actually begin craving more and more water every day. Believe me, you'll quickly come to realize that the water is (more than) fine!

Tips for Wading In

- *Start your day with water.* During my journey to renegade health, I adopted a habit of drinking a full bottle of water first thing every morning. As my doctor emphasized to me, doing so rehydrates you after a night of rest, wakes up your system and jumpstarts your metabolism for the day. Try placing a bottle next to where you shave or where you do your morning devotional. Before you finish, drink that bottle of water.

- *Keep water close by at all times.* Carry a bottle with you in your car (if it's plastic, keep it in the shade) and have one handy in your bag. Make sure you have easy access to drinking water at your office. If you always have water within reach, you'll be much more likely to stay hydrated—and to opt for it over sugary drinks.

- *Add lemon or some other fruit for flavor.* Not only does this vary water's taste, but most fruits also provide an alkalizing effect. Keeping your body properly alkalized is essential to your overall health.

- *Only drink water when eating out.* This practice is good for your body and your pocketbook.

- *Eat more fruit and vegetables.* On top of all of the other reasons to eat fruits and vegetables that we've already discussed, they can help with your water intake too.

Most fruits and vegetables have significant water content. When you eat that apple, banana, squash, or carrot, not only are you getting essential nutrients and fiber, you are also getting water.

- *Replace sugary drinks with water.* The sugar contained in sodas (diet sodas are no better), sports drinks, sweet tea, sweetened coffee drinks, and most store-bought juices is wreaking havoc on our bodies. Sugar consumption leads directly to weight gain and higher incidences of diabetes. Don't drink empty calories. Work toward replacing all of the sugar-filled drinks in your diet with pure, clean water.

- *Drink half of your body weight every day.* Divide your weight by two. That's how many ounces of water you should aim for on a daily basis. As Dr. Don Colbert wrote in his book, *The Seven Pillars of Health*:

  > *Picture a one gallon container of milk and imagine it three fourths full. If you are an average sized person, that's about how much water your body needs daily. If you weigh 120 pounds, you will need 60 ounces of water. If you weigh 220 pounds, you will need 110 ounces of water.*[2]

- This may sound like a lot, but once you start drinking the amount of water your body needs, you will actually begin to crave it. You will end up wanting to drink much more water than you ever imagined.

- *Thank God for the gift of water.* Every time you pick up that glass or bottle, say thank you to God for the living water he is to us and for the physical water he has given us to sustain our bodies and keep them functioning at their best.

These tips for wading in can also be considered your Small Steps to Life. As you begin hydrating your body well, you will feel an immediate difference in your overall level of energy and sense of wellbeing. Don't neglect this important aspect of your health. Drink up, Renegade!

Small Steps to Life
Implement the above *Tips for Wading In*.

• • •

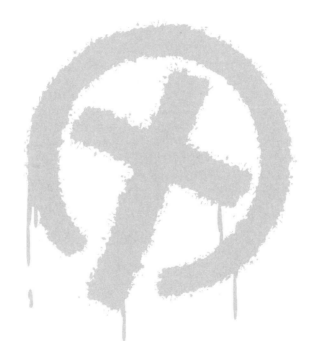

Getting Physical

Getting Physical: Made to Move

If we could give every individual the right amount of nourishment and exercise, not too little and not too much, we would have found the safest way to health.

HIPPOCRATES

So I run with purpose in every step. I am not just shadowboxing.
I discipline my body like an athlete, training it to do what it should.
Otherwise, I fear that after preaching to others I myself might be disqualified.

1 CORINTHIANS 9:26-27

Exercise. It's a word we love to hate, isn't it? Even if you are someone who has enjoyed exercising in the past and understands the benefits for your body, maintaining a habit of exercise is not easy to do. But it is a critical piece of any attempt to get healthy, including becoming a healthy renegade.

In traveling and speaking about health across the country, you have no idea how many times I've heard people tell me that the Bible says there's no point in exercising. They quote Timothy:

> *For bodily exercise profits a little, but godliness is*
> *profitable for all things, having promise of the life*
> *that now is and of that which is to come.*
> —1 Timothy 4:8 (NKJV)

"See?" they say. "The Bible says that bodily exercise has little benefit. I need to spend my time focusing on ministry, not at the gym." I can't blame them for clutching onto this excuse. I used to do the same thing. What I didn't consider, and what they don't either, is that Timothy lived a drastically different lifestyle than you and I live today. In a normal day, just by walking everywhere he went and tending to his business, he was probably more physically active than the average pastor is in a typical two-week period. His life was full of built-in exercise; our lives are full of cars, elevators and desk chairs.

When you first begin your journey to take off extra weight, diet is the most critical factor. Initially, exercise will simply complement the changes you are making to what you put in your mouth. As you begin to drop pounds, exercise becomes more and more important. Once you hit your goal weight (and those new dietary habits are fully integrated into your life), exercise will become the key in helping you sustain your new healthy body for the long haul. This is good news for reluctant exercisers. It gives you a pass to get started slowly and ramp up—which is the wisest approach to a new exercise routine, anyway.

Don't Just Sit There—Get Moving!

The first day I (Steve) decided to start exercising again, I walked into the gym like I owned the place. After all, I was a big shot ex-football player. I had spent years of my life practically living in a gym. How hard could it be to get back to it? Well, much harder than I thought.

There I was, a middle-aged fat guy wearing an old pair of baggy shorts, a nasty T-shirt with a mustard stain on it, out-of-date sneakers and socks pulled up my shins. "Bad to the Bone" might as well have been playing over the loud speaker as I waddled up to the treadmill. I stepped on, hit the green button and I was off to the races—for a whopping five minutes, as I mentioned earlier.

After that first five minutes (of fast walking, not running, mind you), I thought I was going to die! I was pouring sweat and couldn't catch my breath. People around me were watching out of the corners of their eyes to make sure they didn't need to call an ambulance. I realized then and there that exercise isn't a game. My body was being quick to let me know just how far I had let it fall into disrepair. What a wakeup call.

> There will be pain either way; choose the pain that leads to health.

When I left the gym that first day, I was worn out and defeated. But I went back. When I left the gym the second time, I was worn out and defeated. But I went back. Over and over, I went. I understood that, even though it was difficult, I had to turn my health around. My body hurt from the exertion, but what was my alternative? If I quit, my body would continue hurting from the weight and illnesses that were plaguing me. There was going to be pain either way. I knew it was better to choose the pain that would lead to health.

Even though I started slowly, those first few weeks of physical exertion exhausted me. But thanks to God's grace, I was able to continue doing what needed to be done. Not long after, I began reaching the glorious tipping point where it actually gave me energy to work out. I began to feel much better on the days I worked out than on the days I didn't. I was able to accomplish more in my life and ministry because I was taking the time to move my body the way God intended.

You and I were made to move. Our bodies were created to thrive on physical activity. God never intended for us to sit all day every day, overfilling our stomachs and letting our systems atrophy. Unfortunately, sedentary lifestyles have become all-too-common. According to a recent study, the typical American is sedentary for 60% of his waking hours.[1] This lack of physical activity is associated with a number of health problems, ranging from weight gain, to osteoporosis, to cardiovascular disease. Take a look at just some of the problems inactivity causes[2]:

- People who are physically inactive have an increased risk of colon and breast cancer. One study showed a 40% decrease in cancer mortality in persons who were physically active compared to those who were inactive.

- Physical activity helps prevent insulin resistance, the underlying cause of Type II diabetes. A recent study reported that for every two hours that a person watched TV, the risk of Type II diabetes increased 14%.

- Regular physical activity helps reduce the risk of cognitive decline. One study reported that there was a 50% reduction in the risk of dementia in older persons who maintained regular bouts of physical activity.

- People who are sedentary have the highest rates of heart attack. In the Nurses' Health Study, women who were physically active three hours or more per week (half an hour daily) cut their risk of heart attack in half.

- Stroke, which is often referred to as a brain attack, affects approximately 730,000 people annually. Data from the Aerobics Research Center in Dallas, Texas, found that physically active men lowered their risk of stroke by two-thirds. And in the Nurses' Health Study, physically active women decreased their risk of stroke by 50%.

- Bones, like muscles, require regular exercise to maintain their mineral content and strength. Bone loss progresses much faster in people who are physically inactive.

- People who don't perform regular physical activity are more likely to become depressed. Physical activity is a good way to reduce mood swings and helps a person maintain a sense of emotional wellbeing.

- People who don't get regular physical activity are more likely to gain excess weight. One study showed that an hour of walking daily cut the risk of obesity by 24%.

- People who get regular physical activity have a more efficient immune system, which helps ward off various disease and illnesses such as colds and the flu.

Experts agree that the optimal amount of exercise you and I need to get to maintain good health is seventy minutes of exercise, six days a week. If you aren't in the habit of doing much physical activity, then that may sound like an impossible number to you. Believe me, I've been there. Let me encourage you to get started slowly with simple, consistent walking.

Walk for Wellness

Walking is the oldest physical activity known to man. Generations before us walked miles every day and didn't consider it exercise. Walking was just part of life; it was how they got from one place to another and went about their work.

In our modern age of ease and convenience, we've let a walking lifestyle slip by the wayside. Rather than walking a few extra steps, we'll drive around a parking lot for ten extra minutes looking for a space closer to the door. If we would just park farther away, we could save time and get a little exercise to boot.

Most of us don't have to walk much on the job, so we've lost that opportunity, too. Think about Adam in the Garden of Eden. The first task God gave him was to tend to the garden, which would have required a lot of walking. You and I may walk down the hall for a meeting or get up and walk to the coffeemaker, but that's about the extent of it.

Not only is walking great exercise, it's also the perfect jumping off point if you aren't used to getting much physical activity. Walking is cheap and convenient—and it will do wonders for your health. A brisk walk every day gets your blood pumping, raises your metabolism and increases your body's ability to burn calories for up to twelve hours afterward.[3]

That said, you have to walk far enough to make it count. A healthy goal is to get in ten thousand steps per day. In general, ten thousand steps equates to just less than five miles. According to several recent studies, walking ten thousand steps every day leads to:

- A 90% reduction in heart attacks

- A 30% to 70% reduction in cancer rates

- A 50% reduction in Type II diabetes

- A 70% rate of stroke reduction[4]

Getting to ten thousand steps isn't nearly as difficult as you may think. If you remember my health story from Chapter 2, you'll recall that the first time I put on a pair of sneakers and tried to run, I couldn't even make it sixty seconds. That first run turned into a walk around the block—and even that was hard! These days however, I try to run at least three miles most days of the week. Still, on top of that, I have a goal to hit ten thousand walking steps throughout the rest of my day. I wear a small pedometer to track my steps (which I highly recommend; there are many versions to choose from on the market), and I'm often amazed by how quickly those steps add up. You will be, too.

Small routine changes can help you work more walking into your life. What if you decided to take a ten-minute walk after lunch and dinner every day? Just schedule the time into your calendar. Walking for as little as ten minutes after a meal drastically changes your blood sugar level. What would you be doing instead? Sitting back down behind your desk, with food-coma setting in? Sitting down on the couch to watch TV? Those are poor lifestyle choices that will keep you in the grip of ill health. Decide instead that you are going to take a walk around the church parking lot or, if you're at home, around your neighborhood. Take the dog. It will be good for both of you.

As you begin to make walking a habit, you'll naturally think of other ways to work in more steps on a daily basis. Here are a few ideas:

- Take the stairs instead of the elevator.

- If you live in an area where you can walk to have lunch or run some errands, then do it. Limit your driving.

- Have something to discuss with a staff member? Plan a walking meeting.

- Get up a few minutes early in the morning and take the dog for a walk.

- Ignore the most convenient parking space and choose to park farther away from your destination.

Set a goal to get your ten thousand steps in every day. This small lifestyle change will pay huge dividends as you start down the path toward renegade health.

As you feel ready, those ten thousand steps can become the foundation of an active lifestyle that includes other forms of exercise—maybe jogging, swimming, or working out on an elliptical machine at the gym. As you get stronger and healthier, experiment with different activities until you find a few that you really enjoy.

After a while, exercise won't be a chore; it will be something you look forward to, something that brings you energy and joy. Always remember, you were made to move. The more you move, the more you lose.

Small Steps to Life
• Download the audio version of a book you've been meaning to read and listen while you walk or work out.
• Put your work out clothes and sneakers by the bed the night before and take a morning walk as soon as you wake up.
• Buy a pedometer to track the number of steps you're walking in a day.
• For further reading on getting active, pick up Steve's book *Get Off the Couch: Six Motivators to Help You Lose Weight and Start Living.*

• • •

Healthy Renegade Pastor Profile

Josh Hunt
Salem Baptist Church, Salem, NM

I am fifty-six years old and have been working in full-time church ministry for thirty years. I am blessed with great health. Until about three years ago, I had never been to the doctor as an adult, except to treat bouts of psoriasis. However, there was a hidden curse in this blessing. I began believing that I was invincible. Though I never would have said it, I really believed that I was above medical problems. I thought I could live a completely sedentary lifestyle, eat whatever I wanted, gain an extra fifty pounds, and be immune to the health consequences that would come to anyone else doing the same.

Then I did a sermon series on habits that led to writing a book, *Break a Habit: Make a Habit.* This changed everything. Doing the research for this book led me to do a lot of reading on habits, fitness, and diet. As a result of what I learned, I started walking every single day, and I bought a bicycle. I also started using tools like a Fitbit to monitor my progress. I got more serious about my eating habits. As a result, I have lost forty pounds.

I don't think Christians are concerned enough with maintaining a healthy lifestyle. The Bible says that Jesus didn't just grow spiritually; he grew *in wisdom and stature, and in favor with God and men* (Luke 2:52, NKJV). Jesus grew in a balanced way. My question to you is: Do you want to be like Jesus? Then grow in wisdom, grow spiritually, grow socially and grow relationally. Also, grow in terms of fitness. John prayed that his friend would enjoy good health (3 John 1:2). He is clearly not talking about spiritual health because in the next line he says, *even as your soul is getting along well.* Physical health is important.

My biggest struggle with regard to staying healthy is the social aspect of being a pastor. I like to eat, and I like to eat with others. Sometimes this makes it difficult for me to watch what and how much I eat. So I have taught myself to eat defensively. Eating defensively is about filling your stomach with good things so that you won't be tempted to eat bad things. It is about filling up on veggies and salad so you won't be tempted to eat pecan pie.

I also have a goal to walk every day. There were times during the hardest part of this journey when I would get home from a meeting late at night and realize I had not walked that day. Guess what I did? I went for a walk. It may have been a short walk, but I walked. Except for two days when I was sick, I have not missed a day. I try to walk ten thousand steps every single day.

Books on health keep me informed and motivated, and motivation is probably the most important thing. Even if you don't learn anything (you will), you would do well to read books on health for the motivation alone. I also like to listen to audio books about health and wellness. Think about it, listening to an audio book on the benefits of exercise is very motivating, especially when you are working out.

If you are a pastor just entering the ministry, realize that it is normal to gain two pounds per year. Over time, those pounds add up. As pastors, we need to stop making excuses for how hard it is to juggle eating right and exercising with the ministry. We have to lead the way. The reason church people are fat is because pastors are fat. There is an old leadership adage that says the speed of the leader determines the speed of the team. I'd like to paraphrase it and say, the size of the leader determines the size of the team. With small, consistent efforts, you can live a longer, healthier, happier life.

Josh's Advice: It is all about habits. Good habits are hard to make and easy to live with. Bad habits are easy to make and hard to live with. Choose the good.

Before & After

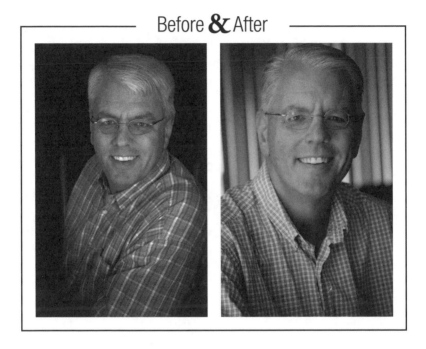

Getting Physical: Know Your Numbers

If you don't know your blood pressure,
It's like not knowing the value of your company.
Dr. Mehmet Oz

For who would begin construction of a building without first calculating the cost to see if there is enough money to finish it? Otherwise, you might complete only the foundation before running out of money, and then everyone would laugh at you.
Luke 14:28-29

As pastors, we love to look at numbers, don't we? We pour over attendance numbers, first-time guest numbers, salvation numbers, giving numbers—and we should. These numbers are good barometers for the health of our churches. Numbers can tell us a lot about what's going well and what we need to work on. They serve an important purpose in letting us know that our ministry is on the right track. (For more on how numbers can help you gauge the health of your church, go to HealthyRenegade.com and download a copy of my free e-book, *What Gets Measured*.)

But while we are experts on our churches' numbers, most of us don't know anything about our personal health numbers. In the same way that the numbers we study week to week can give us insight into our churches, the numbers associated with our physical health can give us insight into the condition of our bodies. Yet, we completely ignore them. Do you have any idea what your cholesterol is? How about your resting heart rate? Before deciding to go renegade with my health, I didn't know either. But now I have come to understand that keeping track of my body's important numbers can help me stay healthy for the long run—and the same goes for you.

Six Numbers to Know

While different schools of thought place emphasis on different numbers, through my personal experience and extensive study, I have found that there are six numbers in particular that you should keep an eye on:

1. Weight
2. Waist Size
3. Resting Heart Rate
4. Blood Pressure
5. Cholesterol
6. Blood Sugar

Let's take a look at each one of these in more detail.

1. Weight

Some experts will tell you not to watch the scale, but I disagree. While you shouldn't obsess over two to three pound swings, your weight is a great indicator of where you are on the health spectrum. Since people come in all shapes and sizes, no one can tell you exactly what you should weigh, but there is definitely a healthy target range for your height and build. Here are some guidelines to keep in mind[1]:

- *Men:* Approximately ninety-five pounds for the first five feet of height and then four pounds for every inch thereafter. So, a 5'10" male should weigh around 155 pounds.

- *Women:* Approximately ninety-five pounds for the first five feet of height and then four pounds for every inch thereafter. So, a 5'4" woman should weigh about 111 pounds.

These numbers may be lower than you were expecting; they are actually about 10% lower than standard weight-guideline charts. That's because many experts are beginning to agree that, as we have gotten larger and less healthy as a nation, our perception of what's normal has slowly shifted in the wrong direction. Most guidelines still put people at risk by reinforcing an unhealthy standard.[2] While these ideal numbers may be hard for you to swallow at first, they are a great target to shoot toward. Even if you don't hit them exactly, you will make significant strides in the right direction by keeping them in mind as your zero-balance point.

2. Waist Size

Again, since everyone has a different build and bone structure, any discussion of weight is a rough gauge. Waist size helps bring some clarity. Here's the key: You can't go by what your pants say. Many of us wear smaller pants than we should and simply ignore the overlap. To get an accurate measurement of your waist size, take a tape measure, hold it to your belly button and pull it around your waist. What is the circumference?

Belly size is an extremely important indicator of health. Having too much fat around your middle greatly increases your risk of:

- Cardiovascular disease
- Type II diabetes
- Colorectal cancer
- Sleep apnea
- Dementia

So what's too much? The general consensus among health professionals is that a man's waist should measure no more than forty inches and a woman's no more than thirty-five. According to Dr. Joel Fuhrman:

> *As a good rule of thumb: for optimal health and longevity, a man should not have more than one-half inch of skin that he can pinch near his umbilicus (belly button) and a woman should not have more than one inch. Almost any fat on the body over this minimum is a health risk.*[3]

I can't overstate the importance of losing excess belly fat. Not only is it one of the single best indicators for almost every serious health condition imaginable, but being overly heavy around the middle also greatly impacts your quality of life. Belly weight zaps your energy and makes it hard to participate fully in what's going on around you. Men, excess belly weight is also tied directly to lower testosterone. Plus, it is the primary cause of sleep apnea and other sleep-related disorders.

While it has become a common look, extra weight around your middle is not inevitable. You can turn the tide; you can get this number down. As you do, your life will improve exponentially.

3. Resting Heart Rate

Before I understood the importance of knowing my numbers, I didn't have a clue what my resting heart rate (RHR) was. I definitely didn't know how to calculate it. But when I first went to the doctor to kick off this weight loss journey, I found out that it was scarily high. What that told my doctor was that I was both completely out of shape and at an increased risk for heart issues.

A high resting heart rate is a sign that your heart is working harder than it should have to in its efforts to pump blood through your body. When that's the case, the groundwork is being laid for cardiovascular problems. A high resting heart rate is a red flag that you are headed down a path to a cardiovascular disorder like heart disease or high blood pressure, if you aren't dealing with one already. The good news is that, if your heart rate is higher than it should be, there are steps you can take to bring it down. The single most effective way to lower your RHR is through regular exercise. As you get more blood pumping through your heart, it becomes more efficient. Over time, a lifestyle that includes regular, moderate exercise will keep your blood vessels expanded and ward off clogged arteries. Reducing stress and losing extra weight have also been shown to lower the resting heart rate.

So how do you know your number? Figuring out your resting heart rate is easy. Find your pulse by placing two fingers on your throat beside your Adam's apple and count the number of times your heart beats in one minute. The best time for an accurate measurement is first thing in the morning. Use a stopwatch; it's impossible to count beats and seconds at the same time. A normal resting range is between sixty and ninety beats per minute. Anything over ninety can be cause for concern.

4. Blood Pressure

High blood pressure, also known as hypertension, occurs when the blood flow in your heart is causing the muscle stress, which is usually the result of narrowing arteries. The higher your blood pressure is, and the longer it goes untreated, the more damage it does to your blood vessels and arteries. Over time, uncontrolled high blood pressure can lead to a heart attack or a stroke.

Many people walking around with high blood pressure don't even realize they have it. As the condition continues to go untreated, the problem worsens, creating heightened health risks and becoming more difficult to turn around. So, it's important to know your number.

When you have your blood pressure taken, either at the doctor's office or by one of the blood pressure cuffs found in most pharmacies, pay attention to the top number. This is your systolic blood pressure. It indicates the amount of pressure being put on your arteries with each heartbeat. Normal is below 120. If your top number is between 120 and 139 you are in the pre-hypertension danger zone. A number over 140 qualifies as high blood pressure.

If your blood pressure is normal, an annual reading at the doctor's office is all you need to monitor it. But if it's high, your doctor may want you to test your blood pressure more frequently. You'll have to work together to develop a plan for keeping an eye on this important number.

5. Cholesterol

Cholesterol is a necessary substance found in the fatty part of your blood. While some cholesterol is helpful for building strong cells, too much of it causes fat deposits to develop in your blood vessels and arteries. Those deposits keep the heart and brain from being able to get the oxygen-rich blood flow they need. Decreased blood flow to your heart can cause angina and heart attack; decreased blood flow to your brain may cause a stroke.

> Genetics may load the gun, but it's your lifestyle that pulls the trigger. —Dr. Mehmet Oz

Cholesterol can be a little confusing because it comes in two forms. There's the good cholesterol (HDL) and the bad cholesterol (LDL). Just remember that the one starting with H stands for healthy. Your HDL number should be over fifty and your LDL number should be under one hundred. The only way to find out these numbers is through a simple blood test at your doctor's office.

Again, high cholesterol is something that can be brought under control with the help of a healthy lifestyle. Being overweight and inactive are major risk factors for high cholesterol, as is smoking. High blood pressure is also a good indictor that you are going to have high cholesterol, so as you work to keep your blood pressure numbers down, you will be minimizing your cholesterol risk. This all works together. Even if you have a family history of high cholesterol or early heart disease, that doesn't mean you are doomed. As Dr. Mehmet Oz often says, "Genetics may load the gun, but it's your lifestyle that pulls the trigger."

6. Blood Sugar

Your blood sugar level is an indicator of your risk for diabetes, which can cause cardiac disease, kidney failure, blindness and a host of other problems. The best time to test your blood sugar is after eight hours of not eating, since food can cause the numbers to spike artificially. This is another number that can be obtained through a blood draw, but you can also measure it yourself through a store-bought finger prick test.

If your (fasting) blood sugar registers above one hundred, then you are considered pre-diabetic. Being pre-diabetic means you're at a high risk for developing Type II diabetes and heart disease. Still, this number is no different than those listed above in that it can be reversed with healthy lifestyle changes. Cutting out refined carbohydrates, filling your diet with healthy vegetables/fruits/beans/whole grains, limiting meat, and getting on a regular walking regimen can all-but eliminate your risk for high blood sugar. When you consider the alternative, why wouldn't you take those steps?

Develop a Plan

I know you are a pro at using numbers to gauge other things in your life and ministry. Now, as part of becoming a healthy renegade, it's time to find out and start keeping track of the numbers that are essential to your health. A good first step is to set up an appointment with your doctor, so you can find out exactly where you stand. Then, you and your doctor should work together to develop a plan to make sure your numbers stay in the healthy range if they are already there, or get back into a healthy range if they're not.

On that note, make sure you have a doctor you are comfortable with; someone you can trust. He or she will be an indispensible part of your journey toward health. You need to be able to be honest with him or her about everything you experience as you drop weight and begin to get your physical body under control. If you don't already have that kind of doctor in your life, make sure you seek one out at the beginning of this process. Together, you will be able to establish and work toward a course of action to get you back in tiptop physical shape.

Small Steps to Life
• Make an appointment with your doctor to find out your numbers.
• If you don't have a doctor you can trust, ask friends or coworkers to recommend someone.
• Commit to monitoring your numbers regularly.

. . .

Healthy Renegade Pastor Profile

Randy Larson
The Vineyard Church, Rockville Centre, NY

I am sixty-nine years old and have been in full-time ministry for fifty years. I have never been overweight. In fact, I have been active all my life and have been blessed with a healthy metabolism. My wife and I have gone through different cycles of food choices over the years, but for the most part I have eaten relatively well. However, several years ago I was diagnosed with high cholesterol. In order to control it, I took measures to eliminate red meat, cheese, French fries, and processed food from my diet. My wife and I also increased our intake of fruits and vegetables. As a result of these changes, my cholesterol was excellent at my last physical. Plus, my doctor said my blood pressure was that of an eighteen-year-old.

Even though weight has not been a problem for me, consistently choosing healthy foods has been. My downfall has always been sweets. One small step to life that I made was replacing soda with water when eating out. That was a significant change because I was a big Coke drinker. My office is filled with empty coke bottles and other Coke memorabilia. Those things now serve as reminders of what I once was. Since going on this journey myself, I have now also challenged my church to put out healthy snacks for our small groups.

Many years ago, I joined a local gym. I connected with a young man in my church who was a trainer, and we worked out together for two years. Since then, he has moved on, but I have maintained my workout program. I do it to stay alive and to deal with the stress of ministry. At five o'clock, four days a week, I leave the office and stop at the gym for my workout before going home. Many times the voice in my head says, "You have more work to do. You can go to the gym tomorrow." Thankfully, I rarely give in to that little demon. Spending time at the gym or engaged in some physical activity is not unspiritual, but rather a critical part of your longevity in ministry.

Taking care of your health is an important part of your ministry. Do not fall for the out-of-context religious line that since bodily exercise profits little, do not do it.

I have three grandsons, and they are filled with energy from the moment they wake up until they go to bed. Becoming healthy has helped me stay fit and filled with energy to keep up with them. Physical health is not something you and I can take for granted. It is something we need to be mindful of and build into our schedules. Poor physical health will limit our effectiveness. Take the scripture to *honor God with your body* seriously, and you will be rewarded with a healthy life.

Randy's Advice: Don't neglect your physical body. It is what people see and what carries you around to do all the things ministry requires.

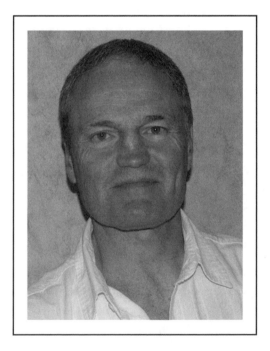

Getting Physical:
Don't Believe the Lies

If you tell a big enough lie and tell it frequently enough, it will be believed.
ADOLF HITLER

When [Satan] lies, it is consistent with his character;
for he is a liar and the father of lies.
JOHN 8:44

Isn't it interesting that Satan's first attempt to lure humankind into a less-than life centered on food? Granted the food in question wasn't a big slice of pie, but to Adam and Eve that forbidden fruit probably looked just as tempting. Well, the devil is nothing if not unoriginal; his tactics haven't changed much. He is still trying to tempt you and me away from God's best plan for us by way of what we put in our mouths—and he is still whispering his lies about our worth and abilities in our ears all the while.

One of Satan's favorite ploys is to continually feed you and me huge helpings of self-doubt and discouragement. If he can make us believe that we aren't capable of living a better life, then he has us trapped. He can control just how much we pursue (or don't pursue) excellence for God's glory. When it comes to physical health, he does everything he can to keep us locked in an average mentality. As I mentioned earlier in these pages, he wants to break our will and make sure we keep driving our bodies further into disrepair.

But you and I know too much to believe Satan's lies. We need to recognize them when they show up, so we can silence them instantaneously and get on with the business of becoming healthy renegades. To help you stay aware of his schemes, take a look at these six deadly lies Satan tells on a regular basis.

Six Deadly Lies

1. Failure: You're not going to succeed.

Have you ever found yourself saying, "I have tried everything to get healthy, but nothing works. This is just the way I am?" Or how about, "I blew my exercise routine (or my eating plan) this week, so I'll just start over on Monday?" These are thoughts Satan is using against you. He wants to keep you focused on past failures so you will think you don't have what it takes to move forward. If he can get you to believe that you always fail in the health arena, then he can eventually keep you from even trying anymore. He's slowly attempting to move you from the *Just Do It* to the *Can't Do It* mentality.

Be careful not to let Satan discourage you with your past. If you have tried to get healthy before and haven't succeeded, then you just need to figure out what went wrong and set out again. Develop a more solid plan and start making the small consistent changes we're discussing in these pages. Jesus promises that you can do all things—including this—because he gives you strength (Philippians 4:13). When Satan whispers lies about failure in your ear, counter his attack with God's truth.

2. Fear: You might hurt yourself (or even die).

We've all heard stories about avid runners keeling over with heart attacks. It happens. Overwhelmingly, the cause is linked to a problem with their diet, not with their exercise, but Satan will use any angle he can grab hold of to scare you into inaction. He knows that if he can get you to believe that exercise can be harmful, then he's won another one to the side of disease through inactivity.

Of course, if you haven't been active in a while, you need to start slowly and do things the right way. But you do not have to be afraid of exercise. To alleviate this fear and be wise about any new exercise routine, make an appointment to talk with your doctor before you get started. He or she will be able to tell you what kind of exercises are best for your body and what you will be able to handle based on your past health concerns and current health situation. Even if he or she puts some limitations on what you can do, your doctor will be excited that you want to get moving.

Remember, God created your body to move. When Satan tries to hit you with the fear of harm, meditate on God's words:

> *This is my command—be strong and courageous!*
> *Do not be afraid or discouraged. For the lord your*
> *God is with you wherever you go.*
> —Joshua 1:9

3. Denial: You don't really have a problem.
As I'm sure you've heard, the first step down the path to wellness is admitting you have a problem. But when you can look around at your family, friends and other pastors in your community who are all as unhealthy or as overweight as you, it's easy to justify your own state of being. You end up thinking, "I'm not as heavy as so-and-so. He should be more worried than I should. Anyway, my weight is nobody's business but my own." Sound familiar?

One of Satan's most cunning tactics is to keep you focused on other people's problems so that you won't look at your own.

One of Satan's most cunning tactics is to keep you focused on other people's problems so that you won't look at your own. He uses this subtle redirection to distract you from addressing the sin in your life. If he can stop you from admitting that you need to make a change, he can keep you right where he wants you.

God, however, isn't in the business of comparison. You are accountable for your own life, for your own actions, for your own weight, for your own health, and the list goes on. Sure, you will always be able to find someone who makes you look good. But when you take your eyes off of that other person and put them on God, your own shortcomings become crystal clear. Taking responsibility for your health and admitting that you need to make some changes is the only way to move forward.

4. Blame: It's not your fault.

Speaking of taking responsibility… it's not always an easy thing to do, is it? In fact, blame shifting seems to be a lifestyle in itself these days. When talking to people about their health, I hear a lot of stories that begin with words like:

- *You see, it's not my fault…*

- *You don't understand why…*

- *There's a real reason I'm so heavy…*

- *My parents always…*

- *My family environment just makes it hard…*

- *If you knew what happened to me…*

I'm sure you have experienced circumstances in your life that can help you justify the condition you are in. Most of us have. But playing the victim is the easy way out. At some point, you have to make a decision to step up and say, "This is my life and my health. I am the only one who controls what goes in my mouth. I am the only one who controls how I move my body. I will not give anyone else or any unfavorable circumstances that much power in my life any longer."

Take ownership of your actions, seek out some wise counsel if you need to and look to God for the strength to help you make essential changes in your life. It's time to break Satan's hold and move into victory.

5. Difficulty: It's just too hard.

Change is uncomfortable, at least for a little while. If you are serious about taking control of your health, you can't be intimidated by the challenge. At the risk of sounding cliché, nothing worth having comes easy. But, rest assured, Satan will try to tell you that this journey just isn't worth the effort it's going to take. When you are struggling during your attempts to exercise, when you wake up with sore muscles, when you feel tired and ready to give up, he will whisper, "This is too hard. It would be so much easier just to keep living the way you're used to." Don't listen to that killer of a lie.

> Refuse to believe the lie that everything must always be comfortable and convenient.

You can outsmart Satan at his game by refusing to believe that everything must always be comfortable and convenient. Stop giving into the path of least resistance and decide to do whatever it takes to live in the body God intends for you to have. You can do this. Yes, it will be hard, especially at first. But with time and sustained effort, it will get easier and easier until, one day, you feel healthier and happier than you ever knew was possible. Aren't you worth the trouble it will take to get there? God says you are.

6. Emotions: You don't feel like it.

This lie starts with small seeds of negativity:

- *I don't feel like getting up early today to walk.*

- *I don't want a healthy lunch. I'm feeling a burger.*

- *I'm too tired.*

- *I just don't feel good today.*

These subtle thoughts lead to poor decisions. Those poor decisions lead to more poor decisions, then frustration and resignation. Beware when they come creeping into the corners of your mind. They direct your feelings and your feelings often determine the choices you make.

You can't base your decisions in life on your feelings; you have to base them on facts. The fact is that if you don't take care of your body today, you are going to pay for it later. Maybe you don't feel like eating well or walking around the block or going to the gym. But it doesn't matter. If you've made a decision to get healthy, those feelings don't trump the fact that you have to take the right steps to get from where you are to where you want to be.

When you choose to do the right next thing—regardless of how you feel in the moment—you will *always* be glad you did. You will never hear someone on the path to health say, "I wish I hadn't gotten that workout in," or "I really wish I had blown it with my food choices today." Whenever I don't feel like being healthy, I remind myself of Paul's words:

> *I discipline my body like an athlete, training it to do*
> *what it should. Otherwise, I fear that after preaching*
> *to others I myself might be disqualified.*
> —1 Corinthians 9:27

I want to live a disciplined, healthy life so I can lead others I care about to do the same. How about you? As representatives of God's excellence, this is not just a personal choice; it's our responsibility. In light of that reality, we don't have the luxury of focusing on how we feel moment to moment. We have to live the way God has called us to live every moment of every day. We can't let Satan's lies sabotage the life God has called us to.

Small Steps to Life
• Recognize and resist Satan's little lies.
• Refuse to play the victim.
• Do the next right thing, whether you feel like it or not.

. . .

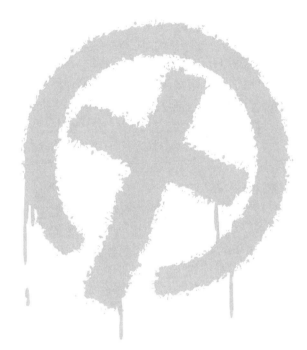

Resting for
Renewal

Resting for Renewal:
How Renegades Sleep

You're not healthy unless your sleep is healthy.
DR. WILLIAM DEMENT

God gives rest to his loved ones.
PSALM 127:2

Have you ever thought of sleep as an essential element of a healthy lifestyle? If you are like most, you probably just think of it as something you wish you got more of; something you can't afford to give much time to. You've likely been guilty of skimping on sleep in the name of getting everything done, as we all have at some point—but that's average thinking. Average pastors stay up too late and get up too early trying to keep a handle on the demands of their ministry. In the process, their bodies, their productivity, and the quality of their work slowly suffers as a result. Healthy renegades have discovered a better way. They have embraced the truth about sleep, and what that truth means for both their health and their effectiveness for the kingdom.

When you and I think like the average pastor, we are inclined to see sleep as an indulgence. We convince ourselves that the hard-core among us learn to push through the fatigue and operate on less rest. That mindset couldn't be any more misguided. When viewed from the right perspective, sleep is the furthest thing from self-indulgence; it's a non-negotiable component of self-improvement, health and wellness.

The Importance of Sleep

Just like your body was created to thrive on certain foods and made to move, it was also crafted for sleep. When God knit you together, he fashioned your systems in such a way that they need deep rest in order to function properly. Without it, breakdown occurs. Don't just take it from me; with every passing year, more and more scientific evidence pops up to underscore just how important sleep is. Study after study shows that quality sleep is critical to good health and to your ability to function effectively on a daily basis. Here are just a few of the specific benefits of good sleep:

1. *Good sleep leads to improved productivity.* When you get a good night's rest, you have more energy the following day. You think more clearly and make better decisions. One extensive study recently concluded that people who get eight hours of sleep each night are significantly more focused and better able to perform tasks given to them than those who get six hours of sleep.[1] A mere six hours was shown to lead to cognitive decline, which resulted in poor decision-making and compromised productivity.

Scarily, the average American subsists on around six hours each night.[2] The average pastor likely gets even less. For years, I tried to convince myself that I could do fine on five to six hours of sleep, but as I became a student of this subject and committed to getting more rest, I realized that I had been living an illusion. I had been compromising my work while telling myself that I was getting more done. That doesn't make a lot of sense, does it? My life was suffering because I wouldn't give my body the sleep it required. Is yours?

2. *Good sleep leads to lower stress.* Sleep is God's prescription for minimizing stress—something all of us in ministry need to do. When you are in a stressed state, the cortisol (your body's stress hormone) levels in your system surge. Over time, high levels of cortisol lead to immunity suppression, weight gain, stomach problems, heart problems

and more. Sleep is one of the primary ways your body neutralizes that stress hormone. When you go to sleep, your stress level begins to fall and your system has the opportunity to normalize. Getting a good night's rest is like hitting a metaphorical reset button on your body. (For more on lowering stress, see chapter 17.)

3. *Good sleep leads to better physical health.* People who operate in the realm of average don't see the connection between getting enough sleep and being physically well in other areas—but there is a major one. Not only does sleep regulate your metabolism and help keep your weight in check, it also lowers your risk of heart disease and diabetes.

You might think it would take years of poor sleep habits for health problems to start showing up. Not so. One recent study simulated the effects of the poor sleep patterns of shift workers on ten healthy young adults. After just four days of insufficient sleep, a third of them had glucose levels that qualified as pre-diabetic.[3]

A Renegade View of Sleep

A few years ago, as I was studying Genesis in preparation for a teaching series, God brought something significant to my attention—a thought that has become a paradigm-shifting revelation in learning to get enough rest. At first glance, the thought seems simple enough: When God created the world, he created the night before the day (Genesis 1:2-4). The darkness preceded the light. While seemingly insignificant on the surface, this thought is transformative when you really follow it through.

In our culture, we consider nightfall to be the end of the day. We work hard through all of our waking hours and, when it's finally late enough to seem justifiable, we fall into bed exhausted. The next day begins when the alarm clock goes off. However, the Hebrew concept of night and day as represented in Genesis is much different, and arguably much more productive. In it, each night signals the preparation period for the next day. Sleep is not the reward for a day well spent; it's preparation for what God is calling you to tomorrow. In other words, tonight is not the end of today; it's the beginning of tomorrow.

> Sleep is not the reward for a day well spent;
> it's preparation for what God is calling you to tomorrow.

This subtle change in perspective completely shifted my understanding of sleep. I began to realize that if God was going to accomplish what he wanted to accomplish through me, then I needed to prepare myself through rest each night for what the following day would bring. My ability to do his work well hinges on me being adequately rested, or prepared, when I wake up each morning. The same is true for you.

Nighttime sleep is the preparation period you and I have been given. It's a gift from the Father. Taking sleep seriously is my way of saying, "God, I want to be ready for what you have for me. I don't want to miss or compromise your will because of my refusal to get the sleep I need to be at my best." Since I have learned to view sleep properly and act on the insight, not only am I more pleasant to be around, but I am also more effective in my calling than I ever was during those years when I tried to function on fumes.

How to Get More Sleep

Still, even with a renegade understanding of sleep, sometimes it's just hard to put down what you are doing and get in bed. We are all guilty of what sleep scientists call "bedtime procrastination." That is, we fail to go to bed when we know we should because there's always one more thing to do—one more email to send, one more chapter to read, one more rerun to watch. You know how it goes.

Just like with other areas of our health, we have to be intentional about getting our sleep to the level that will serve us best. Here are a few tips for breaking the procrastination cycle and getting more shut-eye:

- **Go to bed fifteen minutes earlier.** Most of us have a certain time we need to be up in the morning. Sleeping in isn't an option. So, to start getting more sleep, we have to add it to the front-end of the night. That is, we have to go to bed earlier.

  Try easing into an earlier bedtime. If you suddenly start going to bed an hour before you are used to, you may find yourself lying wide-awake staring at the ceiling until your body adjusts. Instead, go to bed fifteen minutes earlier every night for a month. The next month, go to bed fifteen minutes earlier than that. Keep backing up your bedtime by fifteen minutes each month until you are getting seven to eight hours of sleep every night.

- **Create a bedtime routine.** Parents understand the importance of good bedtime habits. We know that kids go to sleep much easier when there is a predictable routine in place. Maybe it's a bath, changing into comfy pajamas, reading a book, or playing with a favorite toy. No matter the specifics, routine helps signal to our bodies that sleep is coming. As adults, you and I usually lose this practice, but we shouldn't.

  A wind-down routine will help you transition out of your hectic day and into sleep. Don't get too elaborate; just start doing something consistently that relaxes you and puts you in a sleepier mindset. Have a cup of herbal tea or read a few pages of a novel that you save just for bedtime. Spend some time in quiet prayer. Do whatever helps you cross the divide from busy to bed.

- **Do a Big Sleep two or three times each year.** Sometimes the best thing you can do to accomplish more is to get some much-needed rest. That's the idea behind the Big Sleep—a concept I came across several years ago and have made great use of ever since.

  Let's say it's Wednesday afternoon. You are trying to pull things together for Sunday, but because of side issues demanding your attention, unusual family concerns and a slew of other pressures, you are having a hard time wading through all that needs to be done. Your stress level is high; your anxiety is through the roof; you're overwhelmed and so far behind that you aren't sure which way to turn next. At that moment, what should you do?

  Here's what you shouldn't do: You shouldn't keep plowing through. You shouldn't stay up half the night or skip your Sabbath in an attempt to get everything done. Pushing harder isn't the answer. You will just start hitting your head against the ceiling of diminishing returns. That's what an average pastor would do. Though it may seem counter-intuitive at first, your best course of action is to hit the reset button by doing a Big Sleep. Leave everything behind and go to bed for twelve full hours.

  Sounds crazy, right? Trust me on this: the most effective way to clear your head and break the cycle of instability is to do a Big Sleep at the exact time you think there's no way you could afford to. Go home at a reasonable hour, let your family in on your plan, and then steal away for a full, extended night's rest. If you don't think you can physically sleep for twelve hours, use the first part of that time to unwind—alone and completely unplugged from work. Take a walk or read a book, then get in bed nice and early. When you get up the next morning, you are going to be refocused, reenergized, and ready to tackle everything that seemed ready to tackle you yesterday.

Now, you can't do a Big Sleep every night. But if you will adopt the practice two to three times per year, when things seem particularly hectic and stressful, you'll soon learn that the Big Sleep doesn't cost you any time or productivity. In fact, it doubles your time and productivity by giving you the ability to face your circumstances refreshed and clear-headed. All it will take is one or two successful Big Sleeps and you will understand why some of the most productive people in the world have made this a habit.

How Are You Sleeping?

Even when we understand the importance of prioritizing sleep, you and I are terrible at estimating whether we are getting enough. In the sleep study I mentioned above—the one illustrating the cognitive decline among those who only got six hours of sleep—most of the sleep-deprived participants insisted that they were getting enough sleep and that they weren't being negatively affected by sleeping less than eight hours. Yet the research proved them to be significantly impaired. Point being, we are so culturally conditioned to get by on too-little sleep that we are not always the best judges of whether or not our needs are being met. To begin determining if you are getting enough sleep, ask yourself these five questions:

1. *How much sleep do I need?* While there are rare exceptions on both sides of the equation, the vast majority of us need approximately eight hours of sleep every night to function at our best. If you aren't sure whether you need the full eight hours, consider the next four questions:

2. *Am I waking up without an alarm?* If the answer is no, you probably aren't getting enough sleep. When you hit your sweet spot, you may still set an alarm for safety, but you should wake up feeling rested sometime in the thirty minutes before it sounds. If you aren't, that's a sign you need to go to bed earlier.

3. *Am I able to go to sleep within thirty minutes of lying down?* Over a few months, this question, combined with the one above, will help you figure out exactly how much sleep you need. If you know you aren't getting enough sleep, but you are having problems falling asleep when you go to bed, try establishing a wind-down routine, as mentioned above.

If you aren't able to go to sleep because your mind is consumed with worry, learn to turn those issues over to God. Trust him enough to close your eyes and rest, knowing that you'll be better able to face the day tomorrow if you do. One thing that has been helpful for me is to make a to-do list for the next day before I leave the office at night. That way, I don't have to lie awake in bed thinking about everything I need to do.

No matter what you are worrying about, remember, God is going to be awake all night anyway. Let him handle your concerns for a while. As King David wrote:

> *…the one who watches over you will not slumber.*
> —Psalm 121:3

4. *Am I waking up rested and pain free?* When you wake up rested and pain free, you know you're getting quality sleep—and quality is just as important as quantity. If your answer to this question is no, you'll have to do a

little investigating to figure out why. If I had to guess, though, I would say that your mattress is to blame. An old or poor quality mattress can cause disrupted sleep and back pain. The effects aren't worth the few dollars you save by buying a cheap mattress or by holding onto the same one for more than a decade. As your body ages and changes, so do your mattress needs. Take some time to explore what works best for you.

Personally, I saved up a few fears ago and invested in one of the top-of-line memory foam mattresses; it revolutionized my sleep. Not only does it support my body with pressure at the right points so that I wake up rested and without pain, it also keeps my wife and I from waking each other up when we move around in the middle of the night.

While an issue like mattress quality may sound trivial at first, it's not. The more you do to make sure you are getting the rest you need, the better your health, your life, and your ability to fulfill God's plans will be. That's worth the money it takes to buy a good mattress.

5. *Am I dozing off during the day?* If you are dozing off at your desk or while sitting in meetings, you probably aren't getting the quantity or quality of sleep you need. If you are only struggling to stay awake occasionally, then you should be able to address the problem by improving your sleep in the ways discussed here. On the other hand, if you notice this being an ongoing problem—or if you are falling asleep in dangerous situations, like while you're driving—talk to your doctor. Your drowsiness could be an indication of underlying sleep apnea or some other condition that is keeping your body from resting well at night.

Use these five questions to help you figure out the current quality of your sleep, and then do whatever it takes to begin getting the rest you need. Healthy renegades understand that sleep in a non-negotiable component of health. Don't let the sleep-deprived culture convince you otherwise.

Small Steps to Life
• Go to bed fifteen minutes earlier every night this month. • Invest in a better mattress. • Try sleeping with a pillow between your knees to alleviate back pain.

• • •

15

Resting for Renewal:
Ten Ways to Have More Energy

Performance, health and happiness
are grounded in the skillful management of energy.
JIM LOEHR

But those who trust in the lord will find new strength.
They will soar high on wings like eagles.
They will run and not grow weary. They will walk and not faint.
ISAIAH 40:31

I have a good friend in New York who loves to run the NYC marathon. Each year, he spends months training for that November afternoon when he'll get up before dawn to run twenty-six miles. One of his goals is to keep a consistent speed throughout. He doesn't want to run a few miles, then walk a few miles, then run again, then walk the last five, like so many marathoners do. He likes the challenge of trying to maintain the same pace throughout. He has told me on more than one occasion, "Life is a marathon, Nelson. Doing this helps me push through every day of my regular life without slowing down." While I love my friend, I completely disagree with the philosophy.

Life isn't best viewed as a marathon. It's more like a series of short sprints with periods of recovery in between. Think about the way most professional athletes train. They expend a tremendous amount of energy for a season, and then they have the off-season to rest and recover. They repeat that exertion and recovery cycle over and over for as long as they play their game.

These high-level athletes have learned something that most average people don't understand. The body responds best when we stress it for a period of time and then release the pressure for a period of time. I like to call this the *stress and release cycle*. When you and I push ourselves for a season and then allow ourselves to take a little break, our bodies and minds have the chance to recover. That recovery period is when true growth happens. We are able to assimilate everything we experienced and learned during the exertion period, making us more equipped for the next one. When we treat life as a marathon, we never get that opportunity. Instead, we end up becoming progressively less effective and less healthy because we aren't allowing ourselves sufficient time to rest and grow; we aren't operating within the structure of how our bodies function best.

God proved that he takes this concept seriously when he created the world. He worked diligently for six days and then rested for a day. You and I are designed to do the same—to sprint and then to recover. Then sprint again and recover. By doing so, we become better able to control our energy rather than having our energy control us. (To see how the truth of this principle can revolutionize your small groups system, go to HealthyRenegade.com.)

Those of you who are familiar with my work know that I'm a big advocate of time management. Learning to manage your time well can do wonders for your efficiency and effectiveness. It's a critical skill for renegade pastors. In addition to time management, though, you and I also have to become great at energy management. Managing your energy well is just as important, if not more important, as managing your time. More energy equals more productivity. More energy means more resilience to go back to the drawing board when something doesn't work the first time. More energy brings more focus and diligence in the areas of life we want to improve.

On the other hand, low energy has dangerous effects for both our health and our ministries—but that's where most of us live. We walk around in a zombie-like state, in search of our next cup of coffee or a few minutes' rest. Living on low energy means we produce less and at a lower level of excellence. It means we don't have the stamina to address what's important for our betterment, like losing weight and getting healthy. Low energy makes us irritable and less fun to be around. We lose our excitement, so people don't want to engage with or follow us. For those of us interested in being renegades, this is no way to live.

 More Energy Equals More

- Productivity

- Resilience

- Focus

- Diligence

Renegade Energy Equations

Discovering how to manage your energy well will give you the get up and go it is going to take to become a healthy renegade. When you have more energy, you will be more inclined to eat well. You'll want to get out and move your body. You'll put more emphasis on getting good rest so you don't lose your vigor.

The foundation for managing your energy over the long haul is to begin viewing your life as a series of short sprints with recovery times in between. Here are ten other simple tips for maximizing your energy that I encourage you to layer on top of that foundation. Some of these points are covered extensively in other chapters, so I'll just mention them briefly here:

1. *More alignment = more energy.* When you are walking in the center of what God has planned for you, you experience an excitement and peace that goes beyond understanding. That sense of alignment produces energy. The opposite is also true: Misalignment leads to low energy. Take time to align yourself with the calling God has placed on your life each and every day.

2. *More cooperation = more energy.* God created you with certain rhythms and tendencies that are unique to your makeup. Paying attention to what those are and learning to cooperate with them will help you have more energy every day. For example, you're likely either a morning person or a night owl. Whichever way you've been wired, work with that; don't fight against it.

In the same way, you naturally go through a series of energy peaks and valleys throughout the day that are different from the people around you. Recognize when the peaks are for you and plan your highest energy tasks during those times. The alternative only leads to frustration. Figure out what works best for the way you've been designed and then operate within those realities.

3. *More awareness = more energy.* This one works in conjunction with number two. Thanks to the way God wired you, there are certain activities that energize you and others that drain you. These are different for everyone. For example, I'm not good at counseling people. It absolutely zaps me. But I have a staff person who loves counseling others; he walks out of those sessions energized. God created him and me very differently in that area, and we are most effective individually and as a team when we work in the recognition of that reality.

To have more energy, become aware of the things that fill you up and lean into those things. Try looking back over your to-do list from yesterday and putting a plus sign next to the items that energized you and a negative sign next to the ones that drained you. With intentional awareness over time, you can learn to focus on what you are wired for and delegate what you aren't.

4. *A regular Sabbath = more energy.* Your Sabbath day is your rest and recovery period after the sprint of a busy week. If you neglect that recovery, you will quickly begin to feel the wear. Your Sabbath renews your vigor, your focus and your commitment to keep following through with the visions God has given you. Rest always brings about a re-creation. (Turn to chapter 16 to read much more about the importance of keeping the Sabbath.)

5. *Regular exercise = more energy.* As we've already discussed, walking is one of the best forms of exercise you can engage in. And it just so happens that walking will give you an incredible amount of energy. Every minute you spend walking will be returned to you in productivity later in the day. (To read more about the benefits of walking, turn back to chapter 11.)

6. *More hydration = more energy.* Again, as already detailed, staying well hydrated keeps the energy level in your body where it should be. The amount of water you take in needs to match or exceed the amount of water you lose in a day—which is more than you think. Even mild dehydration can alter your energy level, your mood and your ability to think clearly. (For a refresher on the importance of hydration and how to make sure you consume the amount of water you need, turn back to chapter 10.)

7. *More health = more energy.* Of course, being a healthy renegade in all the ways outlined in these pages will increase your energy. But for this specific equation, I am referring more to avoiding the common illnesses floating all around us.

As pastors, you and I come in contact with a lot of people. As such, we are at a higher risk for catching whatever cold, flu or stomach bug happens to be going around at any given time. But there are things we can do to keep our immunities up and ward off the germs that would love to move in and zap our energy. They are many of the same things we need to do all the time for optimal health:

- *Get enough sleep.*

- *Stay hydrated.*

- *Eat well.*

- *Exercise regularly.*

Plus one more big one: *Wash your hands.* Washing your hands often with soap and warm water is the single best way you can keep yourself from getting sick. Wash long enough to sing happy birthday under your breath twice.

8. *Less weight = more energy.* Obviously, the heavier you are, the harder your body has to work to get through the day. Losing just 10% of your body weight can result in a significant increase in energy. Even more reason to shed those pounds and be a healthy renegade.

9. *Less clutter = more energy.* Not only is clutter a distraction to your day, it can actually become psychologically overwhelming to the point of draining your energy. I recently heard about a study that asked participants to perform a task in a neatly organized room versus in a highly disorganized room. Across the board, the participants were less successful in the cluttered room. Not surprising, is it? You and I both know how much better it feels to have a workspace that is clean and organized rather than in disarray. Clutter simply makes things feel out of control, which is mentally draining. To have more energy, have enough self-control to keep clutter at bay.

10. *More praise* = *more energy*. Focusing on the goodness of God will always renew your energy. Take David's words to heart:

> *I will praise the lord at all times.*
> *I will constantly speak his praises.*
> —Psalm 34:10

Allowing the praises of God to be the golden thread through every single activity of your day will bring you into alignment with him. It will draw you deeper into his presence and create enthusiasm in all you do. When you choose to focus your attention on the source of all good things in your life, your energy tank will be continually refilled. (For a more in-depth examination of each of these energy equations, check out my *Energy Seminar* at HealthyRenegade.com.)

Small Steps to Life

- Look over yesterday's to-do-list. Put a plus sign next to every activity that filled you with energy and a minus sign next to what drained you. Going forward, try to focus more of your attention on the things that merit a plus sign.

- Take fifteen minutes to de-clutter and organize your desk.

- Set a reminder on your watch or your phone to praise God for his goodness every hour

. . .

Brian Moore
Crosspointe Church, Yorba Linda, CA

I am thirty-seven years old and have been in full-time ministry for fifteen years. I have struggled with maintaining a healthy lifestyle and weight ever since I started in ministry. Growing up, my parents did not enforce healthy eating habits. My grandfather died at the age of fifty-two from a heart attack. Many of my uncles died of heart problems, as well. Since I played basketball in high school and college, I was able to eat badly and it never showed up in my weight. However, after I graduated from college, got married, and started ministry, I went to the mall to get new pants one day and realized I had gone from a thirty-four inch waist to a thirty-eight inch waist. I had skipped thirty-six and didn't even know it. I was getting fat fast.

Eating is my greatest struggle. I am an emotional eater. I tend to overeat and soothe myself with ice cream. It's how I cope with the stress of ministry. I had to learn that it is important to control my portion sizes at meals. I tend to go out to eat a lot throughout the week, and love to celebrate by eating. Now I am learning to celebrate victories in other ways.

Over the last fifteen years, my weight has been up and down. At this point in my journey, I am not happy with just losing the weight; I am only happy with the ability to manage a continual healthy weight. God has taught me to pray, rely on him and include him in my healthy lifestyle. Once I starting relying on Jesus to help me in this area, the weight started to come off and stay off. I have lost forty pounds, and I currently weigh 220 pounds.

Juggling ministry and health can be a challenge. I have to control my environment rather than letting my environment control me. To this end, I try to have protein shakes available in my office, as well as quick breakfasts or snacks for the day. Now, I do not beat myself up if I'm not in the office at a certain time every morning. I have learned that it is okay to spend some morning time in the gym; I will be a better pastor for it. I make sure that exercise is scheduled on my calendar. That appointment is just as important as any other appointment in my calendar outside of my God-time appointment. If I am healthy physically, then I will have more energy to minister at a greater level.

I have been teaching my congregation that the body is the temple of the Holy Spirit, and that it is important to get healthy for energy reasons rather than vanity reasons. Still, more is caught than taught, so I make it a point to model healthy habits.

Let me encourage you to eat right and exercise so that you will have more energy to do ministry at a higher level. You will not reach your full redemptive potential until you surrender this area of your life to God.

Brian's Advice: You can make excuses about time, however I believe we have time for what we want to have time for. So make and take the time to get healthy.

Before & After

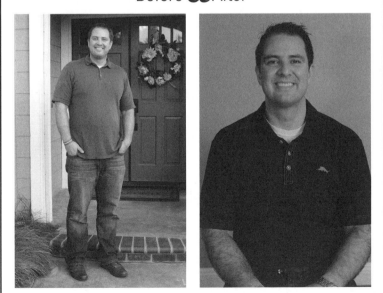

16

Resting for Renewal:
Honor the Sabbath

If you don't take a Sabbath, something is wrong. You're doing too much;
you're being too much in charge. You've got to quit, one day a week, and just
watch what God is going to do when you're not doing anything.

EUGENE H. PETERSON

And God blessed the seventh day and declared it holy,
because it was the day when he rested from all his work of creation.

GENESIS 2:3

I have a confession to make. About two years after I started The
Journey, around the time our New York City location really began to
grow, I was living in sin. I had been living in sin for years, actually,
unashamedly violating the Fourth Commandment:

> *Remember to observe the Sabbath day by keeping it holy.*
> *You have six days each week for your ordinary work,*
> *but the seventh day is a Sabbath day of rest*
> *dedicated to the Lord your God.*
> —Exodus 20:8-10

On a day I'll never forget, a mentor in my life confronted me
about this issue. He called me a sinner for continually failing to take
a Sabbath. He said not only was I ruining my health and sabotaging

my family, but that God wouldn't be able to bless my church any more unless I started taking a day off.

At first, I was furious. After all, I was doing what needed to be done to keep my ministry afloat. How dare he call me a sinner when I was dedicating every waking hour to building God's church? But after I calmed down, I realized he was right—and his willingness to call me out ultimately saved my ministry.

The Sabbath is the key to your future viability. It's essential for keeping yourself physically, emotionally and spiritually well. God didn't slip the Sabbath into the Ten Commandments simply because he thought some time off each week would be a good idea; he understood what we talked about in the last chapter—that continual exertion without regular periods of release would destroy his creation. As Charles Spurgeon put it:

> *Even beasts of burden must be turned out to grass occasionally. The very sea pauses at ebb and flood. Earth keeps the Sabbath of the wintery months, and man, even when exalted to God's ambassador, must rest or faint, must trim his lamp or let it burn low, must recruit his vigor or grow prematurely old. In the long run, we shall do more by sometimes doing less.*[1]

The Sabbath is a twenty-four hour period dedicated to God as an offering every seven days. When that twenty-four hour period is doesn't matter; any twenty-four hours will do. Obviously, your Sabbath isn't going to be on Sunday. A common Sabbath time for pastors is sundown on Friday to sundown on Saturday. Or you may want to take your Sabbath on a Tuesday. The day is irrelevant; what matters is your willingness to spend twenty-four hours apart from all ministry work. For one full day, relinquish control of the universe back to its rightful owner. Choosing to step away, no matter how busy you are or what's going on proves your trust in God's control.

Have you ever had anyone tell you they don't have enough money to tithe? What is your response? My guess is something along the lines of, "Trust God and tithe. You'll see that he's faithful to provide." The reality behind taking a Sabbath is strikingly similar. When people tithe, they quickly come to realize they have an easier time living on 90% of their income than they did living on 100%. (To discover how to lead your members and attenders in a tithe challenge, go to HealthyRenegade.com.) When you choose to honor the Sabbath, you realize you can get more done in six days with one day of rest than you can working all seven—and with more peace, less stress and more effectiveness. When you give God one day, he blesses the other six more abundantly. Trust God and take a day off.

Filling Up Your Sabbath

Part of my original problem with taking a Sabbath, in addition to thinking I didn't have the time, was that I didn't know what to do with myself if I wasn't working. I couldn't imagine taking a day away from ministry work to do… nothing. But as I quickly learned, the Sabbath is not about idling. There are four important elements to an effective Sabbath: Rest, Reflection, Recreation, and Proflection.

Trust God and take a day off.

Rest—Rest can be either passive or active. While passive rest is essential, as we've already discussed, it's not how you need to spend your whole Sabbath. If you need to nap or do a Big Sleep, by all means go for it. But then engage in more active rest. That is, do something restful that grows and renews you. Maybe you want to spend more time reading on your Sabbath than you usually have time for. Maybe you're a big fan of crossword puzzles, so you spend an hour challenging your brain. Whatever it is that works for you, engage in some restful activity.

Reflection—Take time on the Sabbath to look back over the last six days and evaluate how things went. Thank God for what went well. Practice intentional gratefulness. Also take a hard look at the things that didn't go well. The Sabbath is the perfect time to hit the reset button if something hasn't been going the way you want it to. God is giving you the opportunity to fix whatever's not working before plunging ahead into the next week.

One exercise I personally engage in on my Sabbath is to think through the Fruits of the Spirit and reflect on how well I did with each one over the previous week. How well did I love? Did I keep peace or did I lose my temper? You get the idea. Don't miss the opportunity the Sabbath is giving you to evaluate yourself through God's eyes. Think deeply in his presence. That, by the way, is my favorite definition of prayer: Prayer, at its core, is thinking deeply in the presence of God.

Recreation—If you break down the word recreation, you get re-cre-ation. Your Sabbath is a good day to re-create yourself and the relationships in your life. Think about how you can use your Sabbath to reconnect with your spouse or with your children. Schedule time with friends you don't get to see often or reach out to your parents. This is the perfect day to nurture your relationships with the people you love.

Proflection—I made up the word proflection. It simply means to think about the future. Spend time on your Sabbath thinking through the next six days, the next six weeks or even the next six months. The Sabbath gives you an opportunity to do some pre-planning. As you engage in prayerful proflection, God may begin to change what you do over the next six days. You may begin to focus on higher-level activities simply because you've allowed yourself the opportunity to pull away, rest and spend time with him. (For a more in-depth treatment on this subject, see my resource *The Power of the Sabbath* at HealthyRenegade.com.)

You have heard a lot of this before, I know. So had I. You probably even teach on keeping the Sabbath. So did I. But I wasn't practicing what I preached and it almost destroyed me. Are you? If keeping a Sabbath was good enough for God, that's enough evidence that it's good for you and me, too.

Small Steps to Life

- If you don't already have a regular, weekly Sabbath blocked out on your calendar, pick a day and schedule it in. Then take that day off this week.

- When it's time for your Sabbath, focus on resting, reflecting, engaging in recreation and proflecting.

- Ask God to help you trust him enough to make the Sabbath a non-negotiable weekly commitment.

• • •

Healthy Renegade Pastor Profile

Jerry Peterson
First Lutheran Church, Oklahoma City, OK

I am sixty years old and have been in full-time ministry for thirty-four years. I have been struggling with my weight since about 1998. I had always viewed myself as someone in good health. However, my exercise regimen was basically outside yard care. I did not have a real exercise plan. My wake-up call came in April of 2000 when I had a heart attack at the age of forty-six. That was scary! Thankfully, there was no heart muscle damage.

The heart attack motivated me to begin a power walking regimen. I also started watching what I was eating. It worked. I lost weight. At the time, I had been over two hundred pounds, but through diet and exercise I dropped about forty-five pounds. I was able to maintain the weight loss for two to three years, but then I began to get sloppy with diet and exercise again. Since 2000, I have recycled the exercise and weight loss battle three different times, but am getting back on track now.

I am not going to candy coat it for you: it is a struggle for me to juggle the pressures of ministry and staying healthy. I finally came to the realization that I was setting myself up for poor health. The heart attack in April of 2000 was due to stress. It was due to holding on to the anxiety over conflicts and divisions in the church. I was attempting to please everyone. The fear of seeing the church divide or of having people get upset and leave was something I could not shake off. It finally caught up with me.

A major thing that I had not understood or practiced was taking a Sabbath day. Finally, I learned that I had to take time to rest and rejuvenate. I have also learned that a healthy lifestyle provides the energy and motivation to minister and to reach out to others. I serve my church better when I am healthy.

If you are an overweight or unhealthy pastor, please realize that you are shortening your ministry. That heart attack could have killed me. I know what it's like to be overweight and unhealthy versus losing the weight and feeling so much better. I am absolutely amazed at the amount of energy that I gain by burning the fat, exercising and eating healthy. It is a night and day difference! Sooner or later if you keep living an unhealthy life, it will catch up with you. It caught up with me. Don't wait until you have a heart attack to make a change, start now.

Jerry's Advice: Don't forget to keep the Sabbath on a weekly basis. Rest is essential to your success in ministry.

Before & After

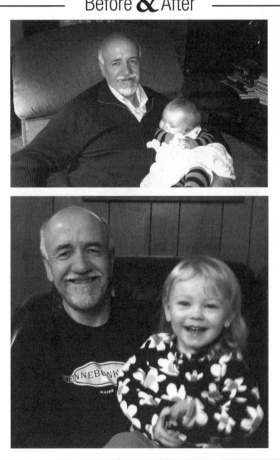

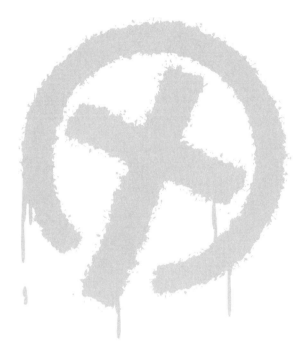

Discovering
Whole Health

17

Discovering Whole Health: From Stress to Rest

If you ask me what is the single most important key to longevity,
I would have to say it is avoiding worry, stress and tension.
And if you didn't ask me, I'd still have to say it.
GEORGE BURNS

In this world you will have trouble. But take heart! I have overcome the world.
JOHN 16:33 (NIV)

There's an old story you may have heard about a man who worked for a major grocery store chain. During an overnight shift, he was working in the store's warehousing area by himself. He went into one of the freezer compartments to grab something he needed and the freezer door accidentally closed behind him. He tried to get out, but he couldn't get the door to open. He was trapped.

Panicking, he yelled for his co-worker who was stocking shelves near the front of the store, but she couldn't hear him. He kicked and banged the freezer door until his feet ached and his hands started to crack, but it wouldn't budge. Finally, he sat down on the floor of the freezer and took out a notepad he had in his pocket. He started recording what was happening to him. He wrote that he was beginning to feel cold and weak. He could feel his body freezing, he said. He scribbled that didn't know if he would get out of the freezer alive.

The following morning, two other store employees opened the freezer compartment and found the man lying on the floor, dead. The amazing part of the story? What the dying man hadn't had the wherewithal to notice was that the freezer wasn't working properly. It had started kicking on and off sporadically a few days earlier, so the compartment wasn't actually at freezing temperatures. But, the trapped man believed it was. He believed he was freezing to death—and the stress his body underwent as a result literally turned that belief into reality. The cold didn't kill him; stress did.

The Stress-Health Connection

Being a healthy renegade goes beyond eating well, exercising and getting enough rest. In order to achieve and maintain true physical health, you also have to learn to handle the stress in your life well. Otherwise, it will derail your other efforts, keeping you overweight, sick, and quite possibly taking you to an early grave.

When you begin to get stressed, your body reacts physically by going into what's known as "fight-or-flight" mode. This stress response causes your heart to race, your breathing to quicken, your muscles to contract and your blood pressure to rise. Your body is literally preparing itself to act in the face of danger, even if that danger isn't physical. When you are in this state often, it wears your body down. Constant stress leads to weight gain, low energy, headaches, digestive issues, frequent colds and infections, premature aging and a host of other problems.[1] Over the long term, it can cause heart disease, heart attacks and an increased cancer risk.

While the physical effects of stress are nothing to be taken lightly, high levels of stress also affect your emotional wellbeing—which is another key component of being a healthy renegade. Stress causes you to lose clarity and make poor decisions. In fact, I would venture that the ten worst decisions you've made in your life were made when you were under a lot of stress. Stress causes you to have a sour mood and a quick temper, which leads to relational issues. There's no margin in your life when you are stressed, so you tend to overreact to everything and hurt the people around you.

Not to mention, stress hinders your spiritual life. Have you noticed that when you are overwhelmed and feel like you have too much to do, your prayer life is one of the first things to suffer? Your time in God's Word usually follows in short order. This creates a vicious cycle. As your stress causes you to crowd God out of your schedule, you begin to lose the sense of his peace and presence—which you need more than ever when you are stressed. This loss causes even more stress, which makes you pull even further away.

Think of stress as something that maximizes whatever is going on in the rest of your life. When you are under high stress, the negative in your life is maximized—health problems, emotional discontent, spiritual distance, relational tension, and the like. On the other hand, when you are managing your stress levels well and keeping them low, the good in your life is maximized. You are able to achieve better physical health, you are more emotionally stable, you have more mental clarity and you are more invested in your relationship with God and with other people.

Stress is an unavoidable part of life, especially for pastors. You are never going to get away from it, so you have to learn to manage it. As Jesus said:

In this world you will have trouble.
But take heart! I have overcome the world.
—John 16:33 (NIV)

With that in mind, consider these three truths about stress:

- *There is no such thing as a stress-free life.* From the average person on the street to the President of the United States, everyone deals with some level of stress. As long as you and I are on this side of heaven, we are never going to be able to eliminate this constant companion—but we can learn to manage and minimize it.

- *Ministry is full of stress.* We have been called into a profession that is inherently stressful. Whether it's staffing issues, growth issues, people who are attacking the church or just the push of trying to get ready for another weekend, stress stays right on our heels. But that stress is continually countered by the victories of ministry—great days when we're able to baptize new believers or reach people in a new way.

- *You are never going to get everything done.* One of the greatest sources of stress in ministry is the never-ending to-do list we all have. There is always going to be another meeting to go to and another budget issue to deal with. There is always going to be another wedding, another hospital visit, and another funeral. If you are like me, you could stay in your office twenty-four hours a day, seven days a week and still not get everything done. That is just part of being called to shepherd a flock.

When you acknowledge these three truths, they actually bring a sense of comfort. They confirm that you are not alone. You are not the only one dealing with high levels of stress. You are not the only one facing challenge after challenge in your church. You are not the only one with a to-do list that seems impossible to check off.

Knowing that stress is a common condition of humankind, and especially of our kind, helps bring it into perspective. The difference in those who allow stress to eat them alive and those who stay cool under the pressure isn't the actual level of stress they are under, but how well they've learned to deal with its inevitable presence. (Visit HealthyRenegade.com for a free download of my *Top Three Stress Management Lessons* podcast.)

Seven Strategies for
Successful Stress Management

Since stress is something you and I have to welcome into our lives and commit to managing well, we would be smart to streamline the stress management process as much as possible. Here are seven simple tips for keeping your stress in check and making sure you don't end up freezing to death in a warm freezer:

1. *Understand the difference between good stress and bad stress.* Yes, there is such a thing as good stress. Small amounts of good stress keep you focused and motivated. You grow through certain levels of stress. The stress gravity exerts on you makes your bones denser and your muscles stronger. When you start exercising, your endurance rises as a result of the stress you are imposing on yourself. When you decide to do something like read a book every month so you can be a better leader, you are adding stress to your life, but it's productive stress; stress that will result in reward for you and those around you. Maximizing the good stress in your life is a wise thing to do. In fact, it's necessary for positive change.

> You cannot always control the situation you find yourself in, but you can control your perception of and response to the situation.

Stress becomes bad when it passes the point of growing you and causes you distress instead. When the phone rings and suddenly you have a problem you didn't see coming; when you realize that you are way behind budget and there's not much time to get caught up. The key with handling bad stress is to continually grow your threshold for dealing with it. Some people freak out at the first sign of a negative issue while others can take the same issue in stride. The difference is their tolerance threshold for stress. Growing that threshold will enable you to deal with bad stress without stressing out. The next six tips will help you do just that.

2. *Get clear on the source of your stress.* Lack of clarity raises your stress level. When a difficult situation sends you over the edge into distress, ask yourself exactly what about that situation is so bothersome. Then, address the source rather than wallowing in the stress itself. Worrying is often just a result of being unclear about your next step. When you can identify the source of your problem, you will usually know what to do about it. You cannot always control the situation you find yourself in, but you can control your perception of and response to the situation—and that can make all the difference in the world in your stress level.

3. *Manage your time well.* There's a major correlation between high stress and a perceived lack of time. If you manage your time poorly, you will always struggle under the pressure of having more to do than there are hours in the day. On the other hand, by learning to manage your time well, you will be able to exponentially increase your ability to tolerate stress.

In *The Renegade Pastor: Abandoning Average in Your Life and Ministry* (Regal Books), I discuss time management in great detail. Most of the discussion goes beyond the scope of these pages. If this is an area you struggle with, take the time to pick up that book. (It will only add good stress to your life.) That said, in the name of managing stress for the sake of your physical health, let me mention three top time management tactics that may help:

- **Don't start the day until you finish the day.** Stress is often an indicator that something in your life is out of control. To regain some of that control, make a practice of finishing the day before you start it. That is, before you start your workday (either the morning of or the evening before), make a list of everything you need to accomplish that day. Sketch out how your day is going to look. Then, review that list, prioritize your most important tasks and tackle those first. Which leads me to...

- **Eat the frog.** As you look at your to-do list for the day, decide to eat the live frog on the list first thing. In other words, do the hardest thing on your list first, so that it won't be hanging over your head and weighing on your productivity for the rest of the day. Otherwise, you will procrastinate on that task. You will let that frog sit on the edge of the desk and blow you kisses all day long while you try to check off other items you enjoy more than frog eating. But getting the live frog out of the way first thing in the morning will lower your stress and skyrocket the overall productivity of your day.

- **Live off peak.** Eliminating wait time in your life will help you eliminate stress. One of the best ways to do that is to commit to an off-peak lifestyle. As pastors, you and I have a certain amount of flexibility in our schedules that most of the working world doesn't have. We can take advantage of this flexibility to cut down on the amount of time we spend doing the things everyone does—like grocery shopping, going to the post office, dining out— and add those saved minutes and hours back into other areas of our days.

  For example, if you are planning a lunch meeting at a restaurant, schedule it for before or after the usual lunchtime rush hour in your community. This simple step could save you thirty minutes. If you have to go to the bank, don't go close to 5:00 p.m. when the rest of the world will be there. Go at a random time in the afternoon and prevent line-waiting from eating away at your schedule. You'll accomplish the task at hand and save yourself a boatload of precious time in the process. Simple steps like these have the potential to lower your stress level significantly.

4. *Practice positive self-talk.* Think of the stress in your life as a flame. When it flares up, you can do one of two things. You can either throw gasoline on it to make it rage even harder or you can drench it with water. The internal monologue you choose will act as one of the two. Again, you can't always control the stressful situations in your life, but you can control your response to them. Part of that is controlling what you say to yourself about those situations. The story running in your head will either make the stress worse than it needs to be or help shrink it down to a manageable level.

You have more power to control your stress than you think. Don't reinforce the chaos in your life by saying things to yourself such as:

- *I'm so stressed out.*

- *I'm just overwhelmed.*

- *I can't believe this is happening.*

- *I'm so far behind; I'm never going to get this done.*

Such negative self-talk keeps the flame raging. Take those thoughts captive and choose instead to see a more positive side of your situation.

The greatest weapon against stress is our ability to choose one thought over another. —William James

Praise God for the work he has given you to do. Praise him that he blesses you with the strength and clarity of mind to handle everything he brings your way. Talk to yourself about how good it's going to feel to eat your next frog. Focus on all that you are getting done. In short, when you talk to yourself, choose your words wisely.

5. *Take mini-breaks throughout the day.* One of the best ways to get ahead of stress is to step back from the situations that are stressing you. When you feel your tension level getting high, take a mini-break. Doing so will slow the momentum of a stressful situation and keep it from spiraling out of control. It breaks the cycle of distress.

Say someone shoots you a not-so-nice email that sends your stress level soaring. Instead of immediately sending an emotionally driven email back or picking up the phone and calling that person while you're upset, step back. Literally push back from your desk and take some deep breaths. Get up and go for a walk in the parking lot. Use the time to pray about the situation. Otherwise, you will just fuel the fire and make things worse. Your mini-break will give you more perspective and allow you to respond from a calmer place.

On a related note, use your transition times throughout the day as mini-breaks—as small opportunities to decompress. In other words, don't carry stress from one meeting to the next. Take a short mini-break in between so you are more refreshed for the next thing coming down the track. Think of your drive home in the evening as a mini-break. It's your chance to step out of the stress and busyness of the day and clear your head before walking in the door to your family. Listen to some praise music as you drive, or do something else that helps you find your way to a more peaceful place. Learn to use these mini-breaks to leave each stressor where it belongs rather than carrying your cumulative tension through your entire day.

6. *Talk to the right person about your stress.* You need someone in your life you can talk to about your stress. A friend of mine, Wayne Cordiero, likes to call this person a lightning rod. Wayne first introduced me to this concept during a Leadership Summit at Willow Creek. Let me explain. A lightning rod is a conductor positioned to

receive electricity that threatens a house. The rod absorbs the electrical current (lightning) when it hits and pulls it away through a wire that runs into the ground. Thanks to the lightning rod, a bolt that could have been disastrous gets easily thwarted.

Wayne explained that we all need to have a lightning rod in our life—a mature friend or mentor with whom we can share difficult situations; someone who can help absorb the stress we're facing and provide some clear perspective. For many years, I made the common mistake of making my wife my lightning rod. When something was bothering me, I would come home and vent about it to her. For example, if I was having a problem with someone in the church or on staff, I would tell her, "You won't believe what Joe Blow said to me." As you can imagine, she would go into protection mode and start feeling resentful toward old Joe. She's human. But in short order, when Joe and I would work everything out, I would often forget to tell her. So even though the situation may have been resolved, my wife would be walking around on Sunday giving Joe the evil eye. Not good.

Rather than making your wife your lightning rod, you should turn to someone more objective to help ground you—someone who isn't in your household. The ideal person for this job would be a friend from another church. Sometimes lightning rods come in groups. Maybe you have a group of guys who would qualify. Just make sure these are people with whom you can share the onslaught of stress you are facing and who are spiritually mature enough to give their opinions in a helpful, non-biased way.

7. *Praise God through times of stress.* Praising God when things are going well is easy, but how quick are you to praise him when you feel overwhelmed? When your stress level is high, practice praising God for giving you the opportunity to grow. Thank him for what he is teaching you in the midst of the fire. Praise him that he is there with you in your stress. Follow the example of Jonah who, when he found himself in the belly of the fish, cried:

But I will offer sacrifices to you with songs of praise, and I will
fulfill all my vows. For my salvation comes from the lord alone.
—Jonah 2:9

Jonah was definitely in the distress zone, but he was committed to praising God and remained focused on fulfilling his calling. As he exercised his trust in the Lord, the fish spit Jonah out and he moved from the distress zone right back into a growth zone.

When you use the strain in your life as an opportunity to worship God for all he is doing in and through you, he will cause it to be a catalyst for growth. By partnering with him and praising him through every stressful situation you face, you will become physically healthier, emotionally healthier, spiritually healthier and be better able to sidestep the negative effects of stress while embracing all that he has for you in the future.

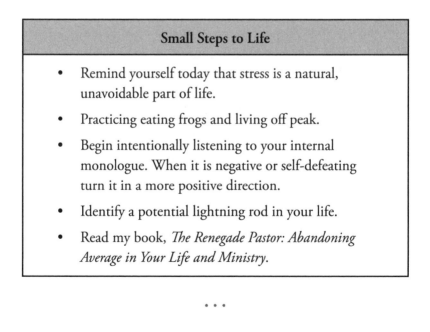

Small Steps to Life

- Remind yourself today that stress is a natural, unavoidable part of life.

- Practicing eating frogs and living off peak.

- Begin intentionally listening to your internal monologue. When it is negative or self-defeating turn it in a more positive direction.

- Identify a potential lightning rod in your life.

- Read my book, *The Renegade Pastor: Abandoning Average in Your Life and Ministry.*

. . .

Healthy Renegade Pastor Profile

Harold Phillips
River Oaks Christian Church, Jenks, OK

I am fifty-nine years old and have been in full-time ministry for thirty-seven years. I have struggled with keeping and maintaining a healthy lifestyle all of my adult life. At the age of forty-two, I was diagnosed with Type II Diabetes. Finally, after years of being up and down with my weight loss, I made the decision to not just try to lose the weight, but to change my lifestyle in the areas of my eating habits and exercise—and to focus on the spiritual aspect of health, as well. Since that time, I have lost sixty pounds and have kept it off. I started this weight loss journey weighing 389 pounds. Praise God, I currently weigh 335.

I don't know about you, but my biggest struggle is maintaining the discipline to walk the walk with regard to my health daily. I finally realized that every food and exercise choice I make carries a good or bad consequence. One of the hardest things about being in the ministry and maintaining a healthy lifestyle is the fact that most of the meetings I attend or lead are centered on food. I have had to learn to prepare ahead of time in order to avoid bad decisions that can cost me later. Also, most of my day is spent sitting instead of moving. So it is imperative that I get up, move around, and clear my head.

Life has many stress points. Pastors tend to internalize issues, especially issues concerning members of their churches. Too often we turn to food to either comfort ourselves or fill in a gap that the Holy Spirit should fill. Learning to control those stress points can make all the difference. I have found that the more consistent I am with exercise, the better ability I have to choose good foods. I currently exercise forty-five minutes per day, four days per week. That helps me keep a healthy balance between food and exercise.

Christians need to understand that the body God has created for us houses the Holy Spirit. We need to present ourselves in such a positive way that people will hear our message. I preach about balance in life. I often refer to Daniel and how he chose to eat differently than the

King's men and how God honored those choices. More than preaching, though, I feel that the changes they actually see in me will motivate the people in my congregation to develop better lifestyle choices.

Leading by example is the best method of ministry. So educate yourself on what it takes to eat properly and then develop a strategy that works for you. You may feel like it is hopeless or like it is too late for you to make the changes you need to make. Let me tell you, it is never too late to start. When I started working out, I could not get off of the floor by myself. Now I can. I promise that you will feel better, sleep better and will be at peace knowing that you are doing what you can to promote a healthy lifestyle for those you pastor. Just a few changes in your daily routine can make a huge difference.

You've heard it before, but it is true: if I can do it, you can do it too. I have wrestled with my emotions and stressors all of my adult life. I always said that I just couldn't do what it would take to get healthy. Well, today I am living proof that anyone can. So, get up, get moving, and glorify God in all you do. You will be glad you did.

Harold's Advice: God has given you a great tool to work with—your body. You should do the best job you can to return that tool to him for his service.

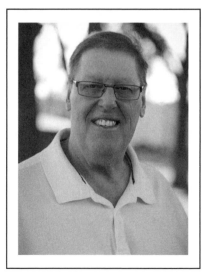

18

Discovering Whole Health:
Maintain Your Emotional Health

I have chosen to be happy because it is good for my health.

VOLTAIRE

But the Holy Spirit produces this kind of fruit in our lives: love, joy, peace, patience, kindness, goodness, faithfulness, gentleness, and self-control.

GALATIANS 5:22-23

As Alex Average slipped down the slope toward too much weight gain and chronic health problems, he also began to have some emotional difficulties. Nothing major, mind you. He wasn't clinically depressed. His emotional challenges weren't debilitating. Still, he knew that the way he was beginning to feel about himself was interfering with his day-to-day activities. He found himself having a harder time bouncing back when things went wrong. He was plagued with a sense that he wasn't good enough and that people didn't really like him. He began to distance himself emotionally from his wife and a couple of his closets friends—not because he wanted to, necessarily; he just didn't feel like he had what it took to engage with them well. Have you ever felt that way?

Physical and emotional health are inextricably linked. It's not surprising that as obesity rates and the related health problems in this country have skyrocketed, so have rates of depression and anxiety. The two areas play on and feed into each other. When someone sees his physical health slipping away, he is at a much higher risk of becoming anxious, depressed and pulling away from those he loves. As that happens, he has even less drive to take the necessary steps to regain physical health so the problem builds on itself. Similarly, someone who is already struggling with depression or anxiety issues is more likely to let his physical health go than someone who is emotionally healthy. Either side can be the catalyst, but both roads lead in the same direction.

Getting a Grasp on Emotional Health

Emotional health isn't quite as easy to pin down as physical health. There are no numbers to measure just how fit you are. That said, psychologists define mental health as an overall psychological wellbeing. It's a combination of the way you feel about yourself, the quality of your relationships, and your ability to manage your feelings and deal with difficulty. People who are emotionally healthy have a sense of contentment and a zest for life. They are able to laugh and have fun with those around them. They rebound from adversity quickly and deal with stress well. The relationships in their lives are good and their sense of self-esteem is strong.[1]

Even though it is more subjective than quantifiable, emotional health is a key component of your ability to be a healthy renegade pastor. When you aren't emotionally healthy, your body will suffer as a result. The negative thoughts and feelings you experience create chemical reactions in your physiology that can lead to weakened immunity, chest pains, shortness of breath, fatigue, back pain, high blood pressure, digestion issues and more.[2] Not to mention, poor emotional health will also make it close to impossible to dive into the healthy lifestyle changes it will take to get your body back where you want it to be. This isn't an issue to be taken lightly. Poor emotional health can completely derail your physical health, your ministry and your entire life.

Issues of mental and emotional stability are often downplayed within the church, but pastors are just as susceptible to these issues as anyone else. In fact, a recent study reported that 23% of pastors say they go beyond emotional instability and actually suffer from mental illness.[3] You and I face spiritual warfare on many fronts every day. Our mental and emotional wellbeing is not immune. Satan loves to attack us through our minds. He knows that if he can control how we think, and therefore feel, about ourselves, he can influence our actions and our effectiveness in this world.

Emotional health is a key component of your ability to be a healthy renegade pastor.

While the majority of us won't deal with emotional problems that cross the line into diagnosable mental distress, we are all extremely likely to experience some level of functional difficulty as a result of poor emotional health. It's part of the profession. Being aware of some of the most common issues that send pastors spiraling can help you and I avoid overwhelming emotional strain. The top three emotional health hurdles are:

- *Occupational Stress*
- *Hostility/Attacks from within the Church*
- *Personal and Relational Problems*

Let's take a look at each of these—and what you can do to counter them—in more detail.

Top Three Emotional Health Hurdles for Pastors

1. *Occupational Stress*—Even if you pastor a healthy, growing church, you will still face your fair share of occupational stress. Such is the nature of church leadership. On top of the issues that come with the day-to-day operation of any church, you will find yourself dealing with your congregants' burdens. You know how it is: People call or email you with prayer requests and some of them weigh on you more heavily than you would expect. When a family in your church is hurting, sometimes it's hard to separate yourself from their pain.

The best way to avoid getting pulled down by occupational stress is to have strong systems in place that will help you deal with it at every turn. Building the eight systems of a healthy church into your structure will eliminate the majority of the stress that comes with the day-to-day details of growing and leading a church. I won't go into those systems here, but if you aren't familiar with them make sure you read *Healthy Systems, Healthy Church* at HealthyRenegade.com.

When it comes to dealing with the hurt that people in your church are facing without becoming emotionally drained, there are a couple of strategies to consider:

- **Let someone else take the lead.** If you are prone to allowing what's going on in others' lives to affect you emotionally, set someone else up as the point person who handles prayer request calls and emails. You likely have someone on your staff who can share this responsibility with you, so the weight isn't all on your shoulders. You may even want to create a simple system for prayer requests to help you manage them well.

  At The Journey, most of our prayer requests come in through our Connection Cards. (For more on utilizing a Connection Card, see *Fusion: Turning First-Time Guests into Fully-Engaged Members of Your Church*, Baker Books.) Our members and attenders write their requests on the back of their Connection Cards and place them in the offering bucket. During the week, various staff people go through them, pray over the requests and follow up with those who are struggling. When something I should specifically know about comes along, they fill me in. Otherwise, I don't see every prayer request. This small step helps me focus on leading without being too emotionally weighed down by the individual difficulties people in the church are facing.

- **Give it over to God.** Even if you aren't the go-to person for personal troubles within the church, you will still walk with plenty of people through dark times in their lives. To protect yourself from the emotional toll that can take, pray continually. Put the burdens of your people on God's shoulders rather than trying to carry them on your own. Let him use you as a source of comfort, but constantly remind yourself and those you are walking with that God is the ultimate healer for all of life's difficult situations.

2. *Hostility from within the church.* Most of the hostility you and I will face comes in the form of criticism. Criticism, if not handled properly, can take a major emotional toll. By calling us (and/or our actions) into question, it usually causes us to default to the defensive—which is not a healthy place to live. But criticism is part of the pastor package. We can't avoid it, so we have to learn to deal with it.

Early in ministry, I discovered that, if I wanted to do anything to make a difference for God, I was going to be criticized often. As a young pastor, this was a struggle for me. I am a people person. I like people and I like for people to like me. Not to mention, I was an extremely passionate young leader. My heart was wrapped up in every decision I made and everything I did.

When someone would criticize me, the criticism had the potential to throw me into a tailspin. Negative, self-deprecating thoughts would barrage my mind. I would try to tell myself, logically, that I would never be able to please everyone; that I needed to take the criticism in stride and move on. But doing so was a different story. Criticism often left me emotionally drained and unable to make confident decisions. I knew that if I didn't learn to deal with this reality of leadership, it would destroy me. The same is true for you. With that in mind, consider these four ways to keep criticism from throwing you emotionally off course:

- **Strengthen Your Foundation.** For you and me, this means going deeper in our relationship with God through continual prayer and study. James tells us that as we draw close to God, he will draw close to us (James 4:7-8). When we are in constant, deep communion with our Father, we are better able to hear from him in every decision we make. Not to mention, we are able to draw from his truth and example when outside forces come against us.

  When I first started dealing with criticism, I remember thinking to myself, "Man, I'm not going to be a very good leader because people's opinions matter too much to me." With growth, I came to realize that my number one concern needed to be to please God, not people. If I was drawing near to him and focusing on pleasing him, everything else would fall into place.

- **Limit Your Exposure.** Limit the criticism that comes across your desk. You are not a trashcan. Negativity will constantly try to push in by way of anonymous emails, unsigned letters or miffed people who want to march right into your office and tell you what they think. If you are serious about protecting your ministry and your personal wellbeing, begin building some "criticism hedges" around yourself. One great way to limit your exposure is to set up a gatekeeper who takes a first look at all of your email and standard mail before it ever makes it to you. I recommend asking a trusted staff member to take on the responsibility. This gatekeeper will become invaluable to you.

- **Run to Conflict.** No matter how much you try to avoid it, situations will come up that call for confrontation. When they do, you have to have the courage to sit down with the person or group bringing the criticism and address the issue at hand. Otherwise, not only will the issue fester in the church, it will drain you emotionally.

  Don't be afraid to confront conflict when necessary. Over the years, I have found that when a pastor is quick to address criticism, the result is positive about 70% of the time. Usually, a simple clarification solves the problem. Still, before you take this step, make sure you are prepared and prayed up. Know what you are going to say and be careful to attack the issue, not the person sitting across from you. Even though confrontation isn't always easy, the end result will go a long way toward keeping you and your church healthy.

- **Focus on the Positive.** When criticism threatens to steal your joy and cause you to get discouraged, shift your focus to all that is right in your life and in your church. Celebrate what God is doing. When you forget to celebrate, you are more likely to let a few critical comments cloud the tremendous fruit all around you. That's not only key to spiritual maturity; it's also key to maintaining your emotional health. (For my free *How to Face Criticism* e-book, go to HealthyRenegade.com.)

3. *Personal and relational problems.* The varieties of personal and relational issues that can threaten your emotional health are too wide and varied to number. Marriage difficulties, problems with your children, a physical illness, financial strain… any of these things, given the right combination of circumstances, has the potential to send you spiraling emotionally if you aren't careful. But you can protect yourself and your emotional health by choosing not to be surprised when problems come your way, seeking counsel when you need it and, again, continually strengthening your foundation.

- **Sidestep Surprise.** Again, you and I are constantly under attack. We face spiritual warfare every single day of our lives. As such, we shouldn't be surprised when things go wrong or when problems show up out of nowhere. Choosing not to be surprised by negative circumstances is essential to being able to handle them without slipping into an unhealthy emotional state. When you and I accept that problems and pain are an inevitable part of life, we can avoid the surprise that makes them even more difficult to deal with. God never promised that life on this side of heaven would be easy; he simply promised to be with us every step of the way.

- **Seek Counseling.** Never be ashamed to seek Christian counseling. Being able to talk to a professional about the things going on in your life can help you process and deal with your emotions in a healthy way. And there's absolutely nothing wrong with doing so—in fact, there are many benefits.

  Several years ago, before my son was born, Kelley and I went through a rough patch in our marriage. We had been married for a while and thought we weren't ever going to be able to have children. Dealing with that reality wore on us. We began to pull away from each other emotionally. Knowing that we needed some outside help, we decided to find a good marriage counselor.

At first, I was extremely hesitant. The idea of walking into an office and talking to a stranger about the details of my marriage made me want to run in the opposite direction. Thankfully, I stayed put. Even though some of the sessions were hard, I can honestly say that the entire process was extremely healthy. To this day, our marriage is still benefiting from what we learned.

Our experience with the marriage counselor made me appreciate the value of Christian counseling. I made a personal decision to start going to a counselor regularly whether I thought I needed it or not. I have discovered great benefit in the process. I expect you will, too, if you decide to give it a try. As I have found, talking to a trained counselor will help you deal with emotions that you didn't even realize you were having. Over time, the process raises your emotional health quotient higher and higher, and serves as a great safety net to make sure nothing sends you spiraling in the other direction.

- **Strengthen Your Foundation.** As I mentioned above, the best way to keep yourself on solid emotional ground is to make sure your footing is secured on the strong foundation of God. As pastors, sometimes we are prone to put our relationship with our Father on autopilot. We confuse doing God's work with seeking earnestly after him. We must be careful not to neglect our personal relationship with God and our growth in him for the sake of our ministry.

Make sure you are taking the time to get quiet before God every day. Talk to him about what is going on in your life. Read his Word attentively and listen to how he wants to guide you. When personal and relational issues come up in your life, don't panic. Instead, lean even harder into the one who gives you the strength and peace of mind you'll need to face them with emotional fortitude.

Keeping a gauge on your emotional health is an important step in improving your overall health and wellbeing. Be on the lookout for the things that can take you down the same path Alex Average has traveled. When you see those things threatening, take intentional action to counter them. Do everything in your power to guard against the attacks being levied at your heart and mind, even as you trust God to do his part to protect you. As you recognize and take responsibility for the state of your own emotional health, you will be well on your way to renegade wholeness.

Small Steps to Life

- Identify a gatekeeper on your staff who can help keep negativity from crossing your desk.

- Run to whatever conflict is threatening your emotional health and your church's wellbeing.

- Find a Christian counselor in your area and establish a relationship.

- Read my book, *Fusion: Turning First-Time Guests into Fully-Engaged Members of Your Church* to learn more about using Connection Cards to help with prayer requests and problems/concerns that people in your church may have.

. . .

Healthy Renegade Pastor Profile

Stan Pegram
BMZ Church, Boscobel, WI

I am forty-eight years old and have been a pastor in full-time ministry for twenty-four years. I have struggled with maintaining a healthy weight and lifestyle since I stopped playing college tennis almost twenty-five years ago. Since those college days, I have had some healthy periods of life and some not-so-healthy periods of life. About fifteen years ago, I entered seminary and that was the beginning of the end of an active lifestyle. I still played a little tennis, but for the most part, I pastored two churches, went to class, studied and ate—all on very little sleep.

After seminary, I knew I had to get back on track. In the midst of full-blown ministry, I decided to challenge myself to drop about forty pounds. It wasn't easy but I did it. I was able to keep it off for a number of years. During that time I began running, and ran a number of half marathons. Everything was going well until I hurt my foot. That put me out of running for about three years, which made it hard for me to maintain my healthy weight.

The biggest struggle I have when trying to stay healthy is the crazy schedule and stress of being a lead pastor for eight worship sites. It is hard to eat right when you are always on the run—and by run, I do not mean actually running. I mean getting in the car, eating fast food and hurrying to the next meeting. In our churches, and probably in most churches, there is always food at our meetings. We call it hospitality. If I'm disciplined, this can be great. If I'm not disciplined, it is trouble!

The stress of ministry is definitely still with me, but with accountability partners helping me out, I am getting back to caring for the temple God has given me to use for his kingdom. Without someone bugging me to stay on track, I have a tendency to get wrapped up in work and push exercise and eating well off of my calendar.

I think that Christians should be concerned with maintaining a healthy lifestyle because first, it is biblical, and second, we have the most important work in the world to do as followers of Jesus. We get to *go into all the world and make disciples.* It's hard to *go* when we can't move. We need to be physically prepared to carry the spiritual load of serving God's kingdom. And as human beings, we are made so that all the different aspects of our being are intertwined. My physical health affects my emotional health, which affects my spiritual health, which affects my relational health, and so on.

We are to be disciples of Jesus. Disciples have discipline. I do not think that there is a much better area to practice being disciplined than with our physical health. Will I have the self-discipline to not eat what everyone else is eating? Will I have the self-discipline to get up early and work out?

Remember that ministry is not a sprint, and it is not a marathon. Rather, it is a series of sprints all connected together. In order to be ready for those very busy, heavy times in ministry, do everything you can to make sure it is not your physical body that lets you down. Just as you work out spiritually by Bible reading, worship, prayer, stewardship and service, do not forget to work out physically. God wants you healthy in this temporary body, so take small steps into an accelerated program for fitness.

Stan's Advice: Seek God, because if you truly seek God then you will have a better understanding of the need for physical health.

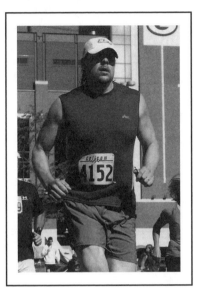

Discovering Whole Health:
Forgive Your Enemies

Never succumb to the temptation of bitterness.
DR. MARTIN LUTHER KING, JR.

Look after each other so that none of you fails to receive the grace of God. Watch out that no poisonous root of bitterness grows up to trouble you, corrupting many.
HEBREWS 12:15

I hate gardening and yard work. I'll admit it. I couldn't care less how green my lawn is or whether or not it looks as good as my neighbor's. Tending the land is just not something I enjoy doing. Since I don't get any pleasure or relaxation from it, I always end up feeling like I could be doing something better with my time. Then I end up frustrated and resentful that not only am I doing a job I don't want to be doing, but I'm also taking time away from other things that are so much more important to me. Oh, and not to mention, I hate pulling weeds.

Weeds are the worst. No matter how often you pull them, there are always more springing up, trying to choke the life out of everything around them. If left unattended, they will devour any healthy growth in their vicinity. A thoughtful grounds caretaker—one much more diligent than me—painstakingly picks the weeds out by their roots, one by one, to make sure they don't have the opportunity to infiltrate the good plants close by.

Still, while I don't enjoy the process of weeding, I do recognize how important it is—and how similar it is to the work we need to do to keep our hearts well-cultivated. If we aren't careful, weeds will begin growing inside of us. Just like the weeds in a garden, they will work to choke out the beauty around them. They can destroy our relationships, our emotional wellbeing, our ministries and, yes, our physical health. Bitterness, or unforgiveness in particular, is a highly deadly type of weed. In fact, unaddressed bitterness is one of the greatest health risks that you and I face as pastors.

You may be thinking to yourself, "I can skip this part. I'm not bitter. Unforgiveness isn't a big problem for me." Hopefully, you're right—but you would be a huge exception. You likely have small weeds of bitterness sprouting in your heart that you don't even recognize yet. Take this little litmus test: How do you feel when people in your church make unfair comments about you? Are you okay with the fact that they talk behind your back about everything they dislike in the church? What about when a trusted staff member abruptly leaves? Do those things just roll off your back? Of course they don't. You may try to say they do, but deep down they hurt. To pretend otherwise would be to deny the reality of your humanity.

Bitterness is nothing to be swept under the rug or taken lightly. A sinful root that produces troublesome fruit, it has the potential to drain the power of God out of your life and mine, and out of the ministries he has called us to. As pastors, you and I deal with a lot of disappointment. We often invest large amounts of time, energy and love in people who end up hurting us. The baggage that people walk through the doors of our churches holding is getting heavier and more cumbersome with every passing year; we can't deal with such hurting, confused people and not end up hurt ourselves at some point. After all, the cliché is a cliché for a reason—hurting people hurt people. Being positioned as you and I are in an institution designed to attract and help hurting people, situations that have the potential to leave us wounded are going to come up.

While in seminary, I became friends with an older pastor who had been in ministry for many years. I was young and on fire for God. I was completely naïve about the problems that pastors face during long years of ministry. While I respected this mentor of mine and learned a great deal from him, he also became a cautionary tale to me. Over the years, he had grown into a negative, bitter man. He couldn't see the bitterness in himself, but it was clear to me. I remember praying, "God, help me stay positive and passionate for you. Don't let me grow bitter." At the time, I didn't realize how pervasive and powerful bitterness could be. Over the last thirty years, I have learned just how easily weeds can spring up and take root in an unexamined heart.

> Bitterness is a sinful root that produces troublesome fruit.

Not too long into my ministry, I found myself heading down a similar path as my mentor. I could feel unforgiveness and bitterness getting comfortable within me. I could sense small changes in my attitude that I knew weren't pleasing to God. Thankfully, through many key personal experiences and a lot of prayer, he showed me how to turn my heart back toward grace and forgiveness.

Bitterness is a troublemaker. The Bible goes so far as to call bitterness a root (Hebrews 12:15). In other words, just like a weed, it lodges in your core, begins to choke the good in your life and leads to unwanted consequences. Bitterness causes unsuspecting, well-intentioned pastors trouble in four key ways:

1. **Spiritually**—When bitterness gets a foothold, it gives the devil an advantage in his schemes to render you and your church ineffective. You can't live in a place of praise, grace and forgiveness when bitterness is brewing—and when you leave that place, you are headed for spiritual trouble.

2. **Mentally**—When you harbor bitterness toward someone, it becomes all consuming. It begins directing your thoughts and, before long, your actions. The person that you are having a conflict with may move across the country or even die, but the negativity you feel won't go with them unless you make an intentional choice to uproot it and let it go. Otherwise, it will continue to grow in your heart and play on your mind, choking out your ability to enjoy the blessings God has put in your life.

3. **Emotionally**—Lingering bitterness can cause significant problems for your emotional health. When you fail to truly forgive someone, that unforgiveness taints not only your relationship with that person, but it hinders your ability to authentically give yourself to the other people in your life. Afraid of getting hurt again, you become more guarded. You start constructing walls around your heart. Inevitably, this leads down a path where trust, grace and love take a back seat to self-preservation. When you are troubled emotionally, you can't engage with others as God would have you engage with them; you can't think clearly and be as productive in your calling; and you are more likely to make poor choices with regard to your health.

4. **Physically**—Bitterness acts like poison in your body. While you may think it's just a heart and mind issue, it's not; its effects run much deeper. The negative emotions bitterness produce are a contributing factor to an array of diseases. According to one researcher at Concordia University:

When harbored for a long time, bitterness may forecast patterns of biological dysregulation, a physiological impairment that can affect metabolism, immune response or organ function and physical disease.[1]

Bitterness and unforgiveness cause specific biological reactions within the body that include adrenaline and cortisol secretions, immune suppression, and increased blood pressure. Elevated cortisol levels tend to cause fat deposition in the abdominal area, which is referred to as "toxic fat." As the name suggests, abdominal fat is linked to the development of cardiovascular diseases, including heart attacks and strokes. (See chapter 12.) Since toxic emotions lead to toxic fat, letting go of bitterness and learning to forgive is not only a weight-loss technique, it could also save your life.

Toxic emotions lead to toxic fat.

How to Avoid and Overcome Bitterness

Your body was not created to house bitterness. Allowing it to linger is like slowly drinking a poisonous concoction. You may not feel the effects at first, but over time it will destroy you. As such, learning to avoid and overcome bitterness is key to living the healthy renegade life. Here are three strategies for keeping bitterness at bay:

1. Expect painful relationships.

Your relationships with other people will be the source of both your greatest pleasure and your greatest pain. None of us is perfect. Consider what the prophet Jeremiah wrote:

> *The human heart is the most deceitful of all things,*
> *and desperately wicked. Who really knows how bad it is?*
> —Jeremiah 17:9

You and I deal with human hearts all day long. Not only is your heart wicked, so is the heart of every person in your family, every person on your staff and every person sitting in your congregation. It shouldn't be surprising, then, that we are going to let each other down. We will disappoint one another. The grace of God is the only thing that keeps hurtful failings and disappointments from happening any more than they do.

Since we are all flawed human beings, we have to learn to expect that there will be pain in relationships. When we think that relationships are going to be perfect and rosy all of the time, we set ourselves up for huge disappointment. When something hurtful happens, we are surprised so we are more likely to respond with anger—which leads to unforgiveness and plants the seeds for bitterness. On the other hand, when we acknowledge that every relationship is going to have its share of problems, we are prepared when they come along and we can deal with them more effectively. We can address the pain rather than turning against the other person.

While pain from our naysayers and distant acquaintances is easier to handle, sometimes the people closest to us are the ones who hurt us most deeply—and the ones it's most important for us to forgive. This has always been the case. Even King David dealt with the relational pain that can come in a close relationship:

> *It is not an enemy who taunts me—I could bear that. It is not my foes who so arrogantly insult me—I could have hidden from them. Instead, it is you—my equal, my companion and close friend. What good fellowship we once enjoyed as we walked together to the house of God.*
> —Psalm 55:12-14

David is dealing with the pain caused by a close friend—some scholars believe that he is even referring to his son. If King David, the man after God's own heart, had to deal with pain in his close relationships, why would you and I think we can avoid it? Let's be quick to acknowledge that pain is part of every relationship, just like thorns are part of every rose, so we can be better prepared to handle it well when it shows up.

2. Choose to rely on God and stay the course.

One of the most emotionally difficult seasons I've walked through as a pastor happened while our church was in the middle of a major building project. Due to a series of unfortunate circumstances, I felt like I was being attacked from all sides and wanted nothing more than to give up and run. During that time, God kept bringing this passage to my mind:

> *In my distress I prayed to the lord, and the lord answered me and set me free. The lord is for me, so I will have no fear. What can mere people do to me? Yes, the lord is for me; he will help me. I will look in triumph at those who hate me. It is better to take refuge in the lord than to trust in people.*
> —Psalm 118:5-8

I wrote these verses on a sticky note and stuck it to my phone, so that I would be reminded of their truth often. Think about the words: *What can mere people do to me? The Lord is for me.* When you are able to keep that perspective, leaning into your reliance on God, hurtful situations with those around you lose much of their sting. He will give you the strength to stand and face whatever you are going through, deal with it as it should be dealt with, and move on with a clear, healthy mind and heart.

As part of this, remember: Nothing gets resolved without humility. As you rely on God in painful situations, you also have to exercise a high degree of humility. Whenever there is strife, our natural tendency is to bow up with pride and try to prove that we're in the right; that our perspective is the one most aligned with the way God thinks. What arrogance. For God to be able to remedy the situation and stop bitterness from seeping into your heart, you must be willing to humble yourself, rely on him and stay the course.

3. Forgive the people who hurt you.

Being able to forgive those who have hurt you is not only essential to your overall health and wellbeing, it's also necessary if you ever hope to experience the fullness of life that God has planned for you going forward. After all, forgiveness isn't a suggestion; it's a command:

> *Make allowance for each other's faults, and forgive*
> *anyone who offends you. Remember,*
> *the Lord forgave you, so **you must forgive others**.*
> —Colossians 3:13 (emphasis added)

Scripture says that you and I must forgive others. There are no quantifiers to be found—just the simple instruction to do it. Here again medical research supports the notion that forgiveness can improve your health. According to a study at Virginia Commonwealth University, chronic unforgiveness causes stress on the body. Every time you think of your transgressor, your body responds with powerful chemical reactions. Forgiving, on the other hand, actually strengthens your immune system.[2] The consequence of not forgiving others and allowing a root of bitterness to grow inside you is too costly to justify. It's just not worth it.

But let's be honest: forgiveness isn't always easy, which is why you and I are hesitant to do it and how it can so quickly lead to bitterness. One of the reasons it's so hard to forgive is because we misunderstand the true nature of forgiveness. We tend to think it is something it's not. Here's what forgiveness is not:

- Forgiving others is not justifying their actions.

- Forgiving others is not denying that you are hurt.

- Forgiving others is not something that hinges on receiving an apology.

Understanding what forgiveness is not always makes it easier to forgive. Given these realities of the nature of forgiveness, who in your life do you need to extend forgiveness to?

In order to offer true forgiveness to someone who has hurt you deeply, you must also understand the process of biblical forgiveness: First, remember how much you've been forgiven. Second, release the person who hurt you. Third, re-establish the relationship (as much as possible). Let's take a closer look at each of the three steps in this process.

First: *Remember how much you've been forgiven.*

Before you can forgive someone who has hurt you, you have to remember how much God has forgiven you. Grasping the extent of God's grace in your own life is the only thing that will give you the ability to offer similar grace to others. While bitterness is a natural response when you've been wounded, forgiveness is supernatural—aided by the recognition of the work God has done in your life and in the lives of those around you.

Second: *Release the person who hurt you.*

Releasing someone who has hurt you means letting that person out of the prison you've constructed in your mind. It means that you stop holding on to the bitterness that has worked so hard to take root; you stop dwelling on how he or she did you wrong. You have to completely hand the situation and all of the emotions associated with it over to God and trust him to deal with it in the proper way. After all, he is much better equipped to handle these things. Once you choose to release your offender, you will experience a great sense of peace and comfort.

As forgiven people, we must forgive.

While you may not feel like releasing the person who has caused you pain, understand that this step is an intentional choice rather than the result of emotion. The only other option is to hold a grudge indefinitely, which is much more harmful to you than to the wrong-doer, as we've seen.

Third: *Re-establish the relationship (as much as possible).*
Forgiveness and reconciliation are not the same thing. Forgiveness is a requirement for healthily moving past pain, but reconciliation has to be considered on case-by-case basis. As Paul wrote:

> *Do your part to live in peace with everyone, as much as possible.*
> —Romans 12:18

You can do your part by remembering how much you've been forgiven, releasing the other person and doing what you can to prayerfully re-establish the relationship, but keep in mind that some relationships can't or shouldn't be re-established. For example, don't reconnect in a relationship that may cause you additional personal harm or expose you to any kind of emotional or physical danger. Be wise. Forgiveness doesn't require putting yourself back in a question-able situation.

If you and I are going to avoid bitterness and all of its negative effects, we are never going to outgrow the need to forgive others. We'll have to repeat the process many times as we move through life and ministry. So one of the greatest things we can do for our health and wellbeing is to make being quick to forgive a habit—a reflex, even. Practice generous forgiveness every chance you get.

> *Then Peter came to him and asked, 'Lord, how often should I forgive someone who sins against me? Seven times?' 'No, not seven times,' Jesus replied, 'but seventy times seven!'*
> —Matthew 18:21-22

Keeping the Weeds Away

Do you have a lot of weeding to do in the garden of your life? Do you have some roots of bitterness that need to be pulled? It is not going to be easy. Remember, just like gardening, letting go of unforgiveness and bitterness is hard, backbreaking work, but it is work that must be done; work that is essential to your health on every level; work that will cultivate a beautiful garden ready to showcase God's excellence to the world.

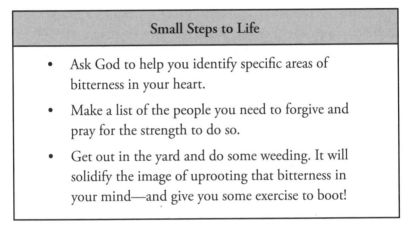

Small Steps to Life
• Ask God to help you identify specific areas of bitterness in your heart.
• Make a list of the people you need to forgive and pray for the strength to do so.
• Get out in the yard and do some weeding. It will solidify the image of uprooting that bitterness in your mind—and give you some exercise to boot!

. . .

Jamey Stuart
Believers Church, Chesapeake, VA

I am forty-six years old and have been in full-time ministry for twenty years. I have to be honest and say that weight has not been my struggle. I think I am genetically thin. But, of course, being thin isn't the same as being healthy, and it doesn't mean that I haven't had to work hard at maintaining my health. Also, as a leader and overseer of a church, I have a responsibility to lead my church to understand the importance of wellness and health.

My biggest struggle in maintaining my own health is in maintaining a regular exercise regimen. I'm grateful that while I work long hours as a pastor, I also have flexibility in my schedule. I have learned to leverage that flexibility to put in place an exercise regimen that is very consistent. Consistent exercise and eating right have helped me to maintain a good weight and to be healthier.

I believe that followers of Jesus should be healthy because it's an important aspect of stewarding what God has given us. In order to live effectively for God, and to make a difference in the world, we have to have energy. Energy comes from healthy living and good management of what God has given us. That's why teaching on health and wellness is an important priority for me. I have a responsibility to teach my congregation what the Bible has to say about this important topic. My church also teaches on health in our small groups. I am passionate about having a healthy church, and that has made quite a difference in the lives of the people in my congregation.

When I first preached Steve's *Bod4God* sermon series in January 2012, one of my members really took it to heart. A woman named Lisa Nowalski lost 135 pounds! I thought that it would be beneficial for you to hear her story and to see first-hand the fruit that can come from teaching your congregation how to honor God with their bodies. This is her story:

> *Every Sunday, Jamey taught from the book Bod4God and for a month I sat in church and took notes. I bought the book and read it every day. I went to the YMCA every day. I removed and replaced foods. I changed my thoughts. God was with me every single step I took. By the end of February I had dropped 30 plus pounds. I hired a personal trainer and started working with her March 1st. By August, I had lost 100 pounds, all accomplished through eating clean, with healthy carbs!*

> *My husband is now coming to church! He was saved years ago but was never active in church. Now my husband is tithing and giving to the new building fund. He said that he feels like God used Believers Church to change me. He is like a new man. So thank you. God used you to save my life and marriage.*

> *God IS the healer! Getting the weight off took all the pressure off my body. I lift weights and build muscle around my problem areas. I started my journey at 285 pounds, 5'9", size 3XL. Today, I am 150 pounds of muscle, and a size four. I pray that the Lord keeps using me. I'm living my **whole** life for him fully.*

Through one sermon series on health, a family was transformed. It is so worth it. I am fully committed to preaching and teaching about the importance of Christians maintaining a healthy lifestyle. I am also counseling other pastors who are currently struggling with their weight.

Even if you are not struggling with your weight or health, I can guarantee that someone in your church is. It is your responsibility to teach the people in your congregation what the Bible says about taking care of their bodies.

Jamey's Advice: Start taking steps today. Even little steps are big.

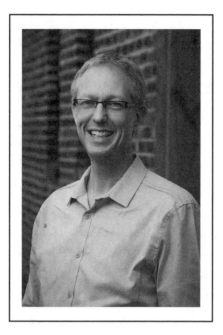

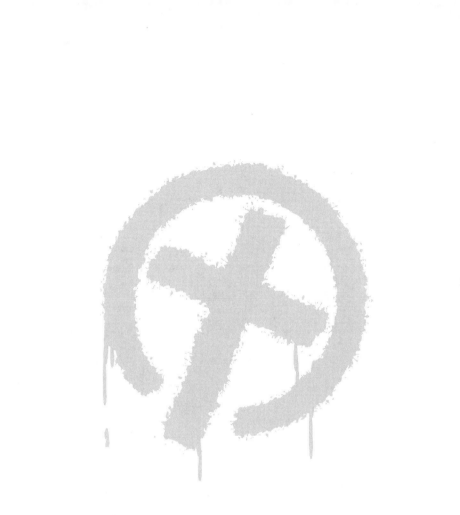

Spreading the
Wellness

Spreading the Wellness:
Shrink Your Church

Good health is a duty to yourself, to your contemporaries,
to your inheritors, and to the progress of the world.
GWENDOLYN BROOKS

My purpose is to give them a rich and satisfying life.
JOHN 10:10

Prayerfully, what you have learned in these pages will give you the
foundation you need to move from average to excellence in your
health; to abandon the status quo of excess weight and disease, opting instead to honor God with your body in a new way. But this
journey isn't all about you. As a pastor, you have a responsibility—an
obligation, even—to share what you are learning with those who
serve alongside you.

When you stand up to preach and look out over the people in
your congregation, how do they look to you? Do they look well? Do
they look like people who are living the abundant life God created
them to live? Do they look healthy? Or do they look like examples
of the statistics we've seen? Are they overweight, struggling with illnesses and so tired that they are nodding off during the service?

These are the people that you have been called to give your life
to shepherding. Turning a blind eye to their physical wellbeing, as
you learn to take better care of your own, would not only do them a

major disservice; it would do the kingdom a disservice, as well. How are they going to be able to serve God fully if they are suffering daily from the consequences of poor health decisions?

In chapter 12, we talked about the six numbers you need to know in order to keep a gauge on the state of your health. Well, now it's time to add a seventh number to the list. This one will help you see beyond how you are doing on the journey to renegade health personally, but also what kind of shape your people are in. This number may be more important to the passion and growth of your church than your attendance numbers from last weekend: *How much does your church weigh?* What would you guess? You and I usually think in terms of growing our churches, but in this regard it's time to start thinking about how you can do your part to turn the tide on the obesity epidemic and help your church shrink.

Shrinking my church was the furthest thing from my mind when I was starting out in ministry. But when I (Steve) began focusing on my own health and wellness, I couldn't help but become burdened by the physical health of my church. I could see my members and attenders struggling with so many of the same issues I had been dealing with. They were fat. Many of them were sick with lifestyle-induced diseases—and they didn't even realize they had a hand in the problem. Worst of all, they were passing the same poor health habits down to their children and grandchildren. I knew I had to do something to change the trajectory of my church's health future.

So I made a decision not to just focus on growing my church for God's glory, but to begin shrinking the people within it for God's glory, as well. My goal became for us to grow through evangelism and shrink through weight loss. I kicked the process off by preaching a sermon series on physical health, *Bod4God*. That led to the *Losing to Live* weight loss competitions I mentioned earlier. (More on *Bod4God* and *Losing to Live* in chapter 21.) Today, we have established an extensive Wellness Ministry to help our people get healthy and stay that way.

Ever since God convicted me about leading my people into more obedience in this area, my church has not been the same; it has been transformed. In total, we have lost over ten tons of weight and become significantly healthier in the process. That is over twenty thousand pounds! Now that is a number I am proud of.

Following the Leader

My church isn't alone. With close to 80% of church leaders being overweight or obese, it's no surprise that Christians are among the most overweight people in America. Take a look at these statistics:

- Fundamentalist Christians are by far the heaviest of all religious groups, led by the Baptists with a 30% obesity rate.[1]

- Young adults who attend church or a Bible study once a week are 50% more likely than those who don't to be obese by middle age.[2]

What a terrible testimony. You and I are called to lead our people into influencing the world around them for Jesus, and all the while we are leading them to destroy his temple at a faster rate than their non-believing counterparts. Through our poor example, we've modeled that health and wellness in this world don't really matter—and that's lie from the enemy himself. Again, Satan is out to steal from us, kill us and destroy us (John 10:10) and if he can lead us to do that by our own hands, even better. Just think what the cherry on top would be for him: if we, as church leaders led congregations of Christians all over the country to their own slow demise by modeling a lifestyle of destruction, and then kept silent as they follow our example.

In the same verse that outlines Satan's agenda, Jesus reassured us:

My purpose is to give them a rich and satisfying life.
—John 10:10

The onus is on you and me to help our people walk in the abundance Jesus promised; something that will never be possible until they discover the importance of honoring him with their entire being.

A Vision for a Better Future

Visionaries change the world. They have the audacity to believe that the future can be significantly better than the present, and a driving passion to turn that belief into reality. While I would never rank myself among the great visionaries who have gone before us, I can relate to them.

I, too, have a vision for a different kind of future—a better future for not only you and me, but for pastors and Christians everywhere. In fact, I have four visions. I'm hoping you will join me in turning each of them into a reality that will change the world for the better:

***Vision One**—That Christians would be the most fit people group in America.* I have a vision of Christians being the most fit people group in America, not the fattest. Wouldn't that speak volumes to the onlooking world? Consider John's words:

I pray that you may enjoy good health and that all may go well with you, even as your soul is getting along well.
—3 John 1:2

As pastors, you and I are concerned with the souls of our people getting along well, as we should be. We want those we shepherd to live faithful, God-honoring lives that shine the truth of the gospel to the people around them. But like John, we also need to begin praying that they will enjoy good health, and that the testimony that comes with that good health will speak volumes in their circles of influence. Not only should we pray for this to be a reality, we need to lead the way.

Vision Two—*That Christians would eat for their health not their happiness.* I have a vision of Christians seeing the bigger picture when they think about their food choices, and choosing to eat for their long-term health rather than their immediate happiness. This begins with learning not to default to the foods they've always eaten and are conditioned to like. There's a wide world of delicious, healthy foods God has created as fuel for our bodies. It will be a great day when we enjoy those foods as much as the manmade concoctions that are helping us dig our own graves.

Vision Three—*That Christians would pray for their wellbeing more than their illnesses.* Have you ever noticed that 90% of prayer requests have to do with health? People always seem to need prayer either for their own health or for the health of a loved one. Now don't get me wrong, praying for the sick is important. We are commanded to do it. But wouldn't it be refreshing if, instead of asking for prayer for an ailment, someone would say, "You know what? I'm not exercising even though I know I need to be. Would you pray for me that I would exercise?" Wouldn't it be refreshing if somebody said, "You know, I don't just have a back problem, I've got a front problem. Pray for my front problem because if I get it straightened out maybe my back problem wouldn't bother me so much." We should work to usher in the day when we can sit in a prayer meeting or receive a prayer request list that focuses on prayers to benefit and maintain the wellness God wants us to have rather than on prayers to get us out of the bad health situations we've gotten ourselves into.

Vision Four—That people throughout our communities would turn to their local churches for help with weight loss rather than to their local secular weight loss program. I don't have a problem with secular weight loss programs; there are many fine ones out there. However, I do have a problem with churches not stepping up and leading in this area. When our people need help getting their weight under control, they shouldn't think first of a commercial for a local weight loss center that they saw on television. They should think of the church—the institution that exists to lead them into honoring God with every aspect of their being. The Creator has better answers for how to live a healthy life than Jenny Craig ever will.

Breaking the Silence

The first step in accomplishing these four visions is to break the silence about gluttony. As we've discussed, gluttony is the acceptable sin parading around in our churches. Not only do we have to address it for our sake as leaders (see chapter 7), we also have to bring it into the light for our congregants. We've been turning a blind eye to its scary reality for far too long.

A while back, I (Steve) spoke at First Baptist Church in Henderson, Texas—a church that was established in 1845. I will never forget a comment one of the church leaders made to me after the service. He said, "You know what? You are probably the first person to ever talk about gluttony from our pulpit." This church had been in existence for well over a century and a half—in what is now one of the heaviest and most unhealthy states in America—and the topic of gluttony had never before been addressed within its walls. The same could probably be said for the vast majority of churches in America, no matter how far back their history dates.

Most Christians and Christian organizations are shockingly quiet on the issue. Just thinking back over my own life, I'm amazed at the lack of attention gluttony has warranted in the believing circles I've been in. I grew up in a Christian home, as part of a Christian church, went to a Christian university and a Christian seminary, and have sat in with some awesome pastors and Christian professors in my life. Never once do I recall anybody ever talking to me about glorifying God with my food choices or my health. Not one time. Yet the Bible has plenty to say about it. Something doesn't add up.

In fact, it's so unusual for the Christian community to talk about this topic, that when I first started addressing it in my church a reporter from *The Washington Post* called. She had received a postcard about the *Bod4God* teaching series in the mail and it piqued her curiosity. When she got me on the phone, she said, "You know, it is not every day you hear a pastor talk about weight loss…." And these next words were especially telling, "…particularly a Baptist pastor." I said, "Ma'am, you are exactly right. I am going to do my best to do the topic justice." To make a long story short, she came to hear the messages and ended up becoming a special part of my weight loss journey. She wrote an article that ended up going on the front page of *The Washington Post*, which in turn produced massive media attention. God used her, and the interest her article invited, to shine a light on an area that has been shrouded in darkness for too long.

Like me, you've probably preached on the Great Commission many times:

> *Jesus came and told his disciples, 'I have been given all authority in heaven and on earth. Therefore, go and make disciples of all the nations, baptizing them in the name of the Father and the Son and the Holy Spirit. Teach these new disciples to obey all the commands I have given you. And be sure of this: I am with you always, even to the end of the age.'*
> —Matthew 28:18-20

Jesus said that we are to go make disciples of all nations, teaching them to obey *all* the commands in his Word. Note the word *all*. We aren't just to teach them to obey spiritually and relationally oriented commands; we are to teach them to obey *all* commands. The Bible uses the word *body* close to two hundred times. There are a lot of commands centered on how to treat and care for it. How well are you leading your church to obey those commands?

> Our silence has produced an overweight, sick, less effective church.

You and I—and arguably every church leader in America—have been disobedient in teaching our congregations what God has to say about gluttony. We have been disobedient in teaching them how to honor God with their health. We've allowed the rampant sinning to go unchecked for too long, and now are all suffering for it. Together, we are facing the consequences of years of neglect. Our silence has produced an overweight, sick, less effective church. It's time to break that silence. It's time to do our part to shrink the church.

Small Steps to Life

- Take note of how overweight or sick the people in your church are. Assess just how bad the problem is.

- Commit to preaching the truth about God's design for our health and wellness.

- Challenge your congregation to organize a potluck dinner filled with healthy, nutritious foods.

• • •

Healthy Renegade Pastor Profile

Kent White
Grace Point Wesleyan Church, Brookings, SD

I am thirty-eight years old and have been in full-time ministry for nine years. Even though I have not struggled a lot with maintaining a healthy weight, I like food a little too much! It's the sweets that get me. I love and eat too many sweets. This is difficult for me because there are always tempting, sweet foods around the church. Plus, there is food at every event, gathering or meeting we have, so my temptation is always staring me in the face. Recently, however, I lost twelve pounds, going from 199 pounds down to 187.

We started a Health and Wellness Ministry at my church, which I endorse and promote. Watching the transformations in the people in my congregation is awesome. I think the key to a successful wellness ministry is finding a leader who has a passion for Christ and a passion for health, and then giving that person the authority and support to run with it. Here is the testimony of Cris Engen, the leader of our Health and Wellness Ministry:

From a young age I was aware of the fact that heart disease affected my father's side of the family and obesity my mother's side. Knowing those genetic risk factors, I have been conscious of good health from a very young age. Through my personal health journey I have developed an intimate relationship with Jesus Christ as my Savior. God's temple is holy, and Christians are that temple.

We all have a gift to offer. God revealed to me that sharing the importance of caring for our bodies was mine. Part of the beauty of having different ministries within a church is that there are options for people to choose from—and when there are enough options, most people will find an area that they are comfortable in. Health in mind, body and spirit is one of those areas.

I do not believe I have ever met anyone who has said, 'I enjoy being out of shape!' We can only be in our best shape when we allow God to work in us and through us. God uses me to share with people that they are valuable to him and that he has blessed them with one body to use for his glory.

If there is just one person who makes changes so that they are able to quit taking high blood pressure pills, insulin, prescriptions for anxiety/depression, or if they can ride on a bus and now fit into a seat next to someone else... those are the victories of a Health and Wellness Ministry. What was once a thought of 'I can never do this' changes to 'I can do all things through Christ who strengthens me!' We hear participants comment on how they are changing from the inside out and how this is making a difference in all areas of their lives.

I encourage you to get a wellness ministry going in your church. Pray for a leader like Cris to come alongside you; someone who has a heart for seeing God work in and through people. We have been fortunate in that Cris has been fired up from the get-go. All we have really done is given her the authority to run with her passions and given her the support she needs to make the ministry the best it can be.

Kent and Cris' Advice: The speed of the leader determines the speed of the gang. As a leader, you are being watched. People will do what you are doing.

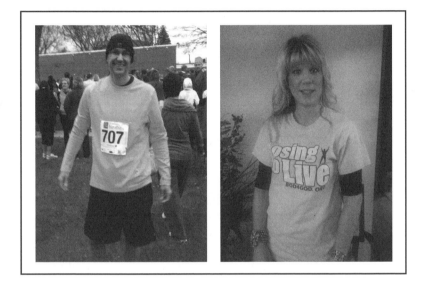

Spreading the Wellness:
Lose to Live

Healing is a matter of time, but it is sometimes also a matter of opportunity.
HIPPOCRATES

I tell you the truth, anyone who believes in me will do the same works I have done,
and even greater works, because I am going to be with the Father.
JOHN 14:12

Throughout his ministry, Jesus healed sick people. After his death and resurrection, the apostles took over the responsibility. The emphasis Jesus and the apostles placed on making the sick well set the tone for how the early church felt about health and healing. Throughout history and into the modern era, Christians have dedicated much of their time, energy, and resources to the promotion of health.

Early believers pioneered the institutions that would evolve into what we now know as hospitals. Christians set up organizations such as the YMCA (Young Men's Christian Association) and YWCA (Young Women's Christian Association)—places where young adults could be active, get healthy and learn about God. In fact, the Y's creator claimed that it was founded to put Christian principles into practice by helping people develop a healthy "body, mind and spirit."[1]

Following Jesus' example, Christians used to be on the front lines of encouraging physical wellbeing. Unfortunately, we have dropped the ball in more recent decades. We stepped back and that silence crept in. Somehow we went from leading the charge of caring for people's physical needs to ignoring issues of health altogether, as we've discussed. This turn likely started when the idea of the Social Gospel was on the rise in the early 20th century. During this movement, many Christians became overly focused on an array of pressing social issues, including health, at the expense of sharing the gospel. As a result, many church leaders reacted strongly by shifting the attention back to the gospel and eschewing any real connection with social issues. The two focuses became mutually exclusive.

The thing is, you and I do not have to choose one over the other. Jesus didn't intend for us to. Not only can we carry the gospel into the world, we can also provide a place where people's physical needs are addressed and cared for. In fact, based on Jesus' example and the church's history, that's exactly what we should be doing. We do a disservice to our people and to the greater community when we delegate all issues of health and wellness to outside organizations.

Today, the people in our churches are sick. They don't understand the consequences of their poor lifestyle choices, or see the self-induced nature of so many of their struggles. Like Jesus, his apostles and the early church, we need to be on the forefront of helping our people get well. It is time to get back to carrying out the work that our predecessors modeled for us, and to get intentional about ministering to the physical health of those around us even as we are ministering to their spiritual health. After all, isn't that what Jesus would want us to do?

Top Three Reasons to Establish a Wellness Ministry in Your Church

The single most effective thing you and I can do to help our congregations get back on the path to God-glorifying health is to set up a strong health and wellness ministry. Without one, we leave them with no real opportunity to build a healthy lifestyle on the only foundation that will sustain it for the long term—an understanding of God's desire and plan for their physical wellness. Take a look at three convincing reasons why you, and every pastor who cares for the full spectrum of his peoples' needs, should set up a wellness ministry:

1. Establish a wellness ministry to encourage your congregation.

In 1 Thessalonians 5:23, Paul wrote:

> *Now may the God of peace make you holy in every way, and may your whole spirit and soul and body be kept blameless until our Lord Jesus Christ comes again.*

Paul said that the whole spirit, soul and body should be blameless. In other words, we are to be sanctified, or set apart, completely. As long as the people in our churches are following the wisdom of the world in their health choices, they will never be fully sanctified. They will remain overweight, sick and frustrated with their attempts to change. But as we begin charting the course together, we can give them a new outlook on how and why to care for their bodies well. We can give them the encouragement and accountability they need to live God-honoring lives in the area of physical wellness.

2. Establish a wellness ministry to evangelize your community.

Paul also wrote:

> *When I am with those who are weak, I share their weakness, for I want to bring the weak to Christ. Yes, I try to find common ground with everyone, doing everything I can to save some. I do everything to spread the Good News and share in its blessings.*
> —1 Corinthians 9:22-23

People in our greater communities are struggling, as well. We have an incredible opportunity to invite them into our gatherings and help them discover how to better care for their bodies.

There is such a need for truth in the area of health that people from every walk of life will come to your church if they think you have some answers. Discussions about wellness and weight loss will attract people who are far from God. In our church, we've had many atheists come to our program. We've had Muslims participate. I will never forget one Muslim lady coming up to me saying, "Okay, I have looked at your program, and I will do everything you suggest here, except memorize the verses." That woman ended up bringing about a dozen Muslims to our church specifically for our wellness ministry. These are people who would never come to hear me preach on anything else, but they became willing to admit that the Bible could teach them something about finding better health. That's a great start.

3. *Establish a wellness ministry to help people commit to an ongoing healthy lifestyle.*

Early in these pages, we looked at the reminder in 1 Corinthians that our bodies were made for God and that he cares about them:

> *[Our bodies] **were made for the Lord**,*
> *and the Lord cares about our bodies.*
> —1 Corinthians 6:13

That paradigm-shifting reality will be an important key in helping your people adopt an ongoing, healthy lifestyle. It gives them a *why* that makes the *what* well worth it. One of the biggest reasons people fail to stick with weight loss and health goals is that they think short-term. They don't develop a new lifestyle—and that's because their *why* isn't substantial enough.

By tying your people's health and wellness goals to the truth that God wants to do more in them and through them than they can imagine, they will be better able to commit to getting in good physical shape for the long haul. After all, not one of them, once walking in that understanding, will want to miss out on the best that God has in store simply because their body isn't in good enough shape to take advantage of it. With a little understanding and some hard work, they will be able to cooperate with him to fulfill his purposes for them on this earth—and if that's not worth some simple, ongoing lifestyle changes then I don't know what is!

Three Common Questions from Pastors

When it comes to actually setting up a wellness ministry, there are three common concerns that most pastors have:

Question One*—Where will I find the volunteers to run this ministry?*

If you struggle finding volunteers for the other ministries in your church, you may be hesitant to start a wellness ministry for fear that you won't have anyone to run it. Let me assure you, health and wellness is an area that certain people will become very excited about. If you do a good job casting the vision, the right people will latch on and want to run with it. There are people sitting in your church right now who aren't serving anywhere else, but who will get very excited to jump into this ministry. And as your church gets healthier together, more and more people will want to give back by volunteering with the ministry, as well.

Question Two*—Will people be offended if I talk about them being overweight?*

Early on, this question was a major concern of mine, too. I was terrified of what people would think if I said they needed to lose weight.

I was afraid that the heaviest people in the church would feel like they were being exposed or having a finger pointed in their direction. After much experience, I have come to realize that people are not offended. Rather, they are relieved to have such a personal struggle brought into the light and dealt with in an honest, biblical way. Our fear of what others may think is just a tactic of the enemy to keep us silent on this issue. When something is scripturally sound, the people sitting in your church aren't generally going to take offense. They are going to welcome the truth.

Question Three—*Shouldn't I lose weight before I start trying to minister about health and wellness?*

Since close to 80% of pastors are overweight or obese, it's likely that you fall into that category. If you do, you may be tempted to think that you need to get yourself in shape before you can stand up and preach to others on the topic. While I understand the thinking, losing the weight you need to lose is not a prerequisite to ministering effectively to others about health and wellness. Your public admission of your own struggles will actually help both you and your church members begin the process of change. Your transparency will heighten the importance of the issue and inspire them to join you in this journey.

People don't want a perfect pastor; they want someone who is real, vulnerable, and willing to admit his own shortcomings. When you choose to acknowledge that you need just as much help as the people sitting in the pews, they will trust you more and relate to you better. Rather than trying to get your health ducks in a row before you start bringing this topic to light, just jump in and do it. Lose your weight in front of their eyes, as they lose their weight in front of yours. There's no better way to break the silence and begin to reclaim our churches and our bodies for God's best.

If you and I do not lead in this vital area, the long-term effectiveness of the church could be severely damaged. Satan is hoping that we will sit back and continue to do nothing so that God's people will keep getting bigger and unhealthier, becoming less able to shine the light of the gospel to the world.

Teaching Your Church How to Lose to Live

One of the best ways to lead your congregation toward a healthier lifestyle is to have a specific game plan in place that can operate under the umbrella of your wellness ministry. As mentioned, after I (Steve) began focusing on my own health, I put together a sermon series called *Bod4God* to launch my church's health and wellness ministry. The content of that sermon series quickly gained momentum and became a way of life for the people in my church. Shortly thereafter, it also became the basis of my first book, *Bod4God: The Four Keys to Weight Loss*. Since its inception, *Bod4God* has helped countless people take control of their health and step into more abundant life.

If you are interested in using *Bod4God* in your church, here are four ways you can get started:

1. Introduce *Bod4God* as a sermon series. You can use the *Bod4God* sermon series as a way to jump-start your congregation's excitement about health and wellness. It also serves as a great attraction series for the wider community. Before our kick-off of *Bod4God*, we made sure to promote it heavily. Still, I didn't know for sure that people would show up for a series on health. But show up they did! We had record attendance on the first Sunday of the series.

On that day, I stood before our congregation and told them that I believed we were one of the most spiritually healthy churches anywhere in America, but that we were not one of the most physically healthy. I let them know that I was committed not only helping them be spiritually fit, but also to helping them be physically fit. I stressed that if they didn't have the temple to support the spiritual activities that God wanted to do in their lives, then they could never live up to their God-given potential. That challenge resonated, and our congregation embraced the call to better health.

I encourage you to start praying about whether or not God would have you add the *Bod4God* messages to your preaching calendar. If you are interested in hearing or using them, go to Bod4God. org. You might be surprised to see what God does in your congregation through strong teaching on his plan for their health.

2. Use *Bod4God* as a small groups book. *Bod4God* is an ideal small groups book. Working through the material with others on the same journey provides people with a healthy environment for sharing their ideas, struggles and victories as they take hold of this new lifestyle. Life-long bonds are formed and miracles happen when people start joining together to get healthy. You may want to implement a few *Bod4God* small groups in your church whether you are also preaching the message series or not.

3. Introduce *Bod4God* as a devotional book. Many people prefer to use the *Bod4God* book as a devotional. They like working through the material on their own, at their own pace. Reading the book in this way gives them the opportunity to get quiet before God, praying and meditating on what they are learning and how they can better care for themselves.

4. Implement *Bod4God*'s weight-loss competition aspect, *Losing to Live*. *Losing to Live* is the weight-loss competition arm of the *Bod4God* program. It is one of the most effective avenues for getting people to embrace a commitment to renewed health. The friendly competition offers people an opportunity to pursue their health goals in a fun and supportive environment. As they work together with their team to get healthier, significant life change happens. I have seen not only my own church, but also churches across the country, transformed by these competitions. For a step-by-step plan on how to start a *Losing to Live* campaign in your church, see Appendix A or go to Bod4God.org.

Now is the Time

The time has come for you and me to abandon average and go renegade with our health. And the time has also come for us to lead those God has entrusted to our care to do the same. The *Bod4God* program can provide the framework to do just that, but you and I have to step up and lead in a way that people will want to follow. We have to get excited about changing our own lives and helping those around us change theirs, all for the glory of the One who formed us and gave us breath.

> Let's transform the church into a healthy body made up of healthy renegade people, ready to walk in step with God's highest design for their lives.

Let's start educating our people well and giving them the tools they need to begin honoring God with their whole bodies. Are you up for the challenge, Healthy Renegade Pastor? Let's transform the church into a healthy body made up of healthy renegade people, ready to walk in step with God's highest design for their lives. As you and I do our part to make that happen, he will meet us in the process and reclaim his creation's health one person at a time!

Small Steps to Life

- Take full advantage of the resources at HealthyRenegade.com and Bod4God.org, including access to healthy living messages and the *Losing to Live* starter kit.

- Read my book, *Connect: How to Double Your Number of Volunteers* (Baker Books 2012) for more practical guidance on creating a new ministry and recruiting eager volunteers.

- Read Steve's book *Bod4God* and sign up for his free resources and newsletter on the subject at Bod4God.org.

- Reach out to members of your church who are doctors, nurses, nutritionists, personal trainers, or other types of health professionals and ask them to volunteer in your new wellness ministry.

- Invest in a professional grade, digital scale and challenge your people to a twelve-week weight loss competition. For more details on organizing the competition, see Appendix A and visit Bod4God.org.

• • •

Spreading the Wellness: Choose Life

To live is to choose. But to choose well, you must know who you are
and what you stand for, where you want to go and why you want to get there.
KOFI ANNAN

Today I have given you the choice between life and death, between blessings and
curses. Now I call on heaven and earth to witness the choice you make.
Oh, that you would choose life, so that you and your descendants might live!
DEUTERONOMY 30:19

As pastors, you and I are driven by the concept of life. We advise
people on how to live it, caution them not to ruin it, and help them
pick up the pieces when it does go wrong. We celebrate with excited
families at the beginning of it, and mourn with the brokenhearted
when it comes to an end. We teach people how to take hold of life
that's eternal, while showing them how to walk in more abundant life
here on earth. When you get down to the core of what we do day in
and day out, our calling is to promote life.

Within that calling, most of our time is spent focusing on the
spiritual and eternal aspects of life—and that's okay; it should be. My
prayer, however, is that through these pages, you have become aware
of the importance of giving attention to the way we interact with the
world physically, as well. As we have seen, God truly cares about how

you and I walk through our days here on earth and how we choose to treat the vessels he has given us specifically for this journey.

While we are all looking eagerly toward the day when we will meet Jesus, we can't neglect the importance of maximizing the time he has given us in this life for its full benefit. What you and I do today will affect not only our own eternities, but those of other people. How well or how poorly we choose to treat our bodies right now will shape the influence we can have on those around us and the impact we will make for God's kingdom. As we close this book and our time together, I challenge you: Choose life. Choose blessing. Choose health and wellbeing over cursing, sickness and death. That's the only way to be able to fulfill the purposes that God has designed for you. Here are four key steps to help you get started.

Four Steps to Choosing Life

1. Stop procrastinating. Procrastination derails more good health intentions than just about anything else. We always think we can eat whatever we want to today because we are going to start losing weight tomorrow. We allow ourselves to gorge during one season by promising ourselves that we are going to "get serious" the next. Can you relate? The problem is that tomorrow always becomes today and, when it does, there's inevitably something else giving us an excuse to wait until the next tomorrow to get started. As the book of Proverbs warns:

> *Don't brag about tomorrow, since you don't*
> *know what the day will bring.*
> —Proverbs 27:1

Not only may tomorrow bring circumstances that will make it harder to start a new healthy lifestyle, tomorrow may actually be too late. Heart attacks happen in the blink of an eye. There are seed-lings of diseases lurking inside each one of us right now that have the potential to come to fruition and overtake us if we persist in an unhealthy lifestyle. You and I don't know when it's going to be too late to turn back; we can't afford to keep procrastinating.

2. Invest in yourself. I know you are committed to investing in others, but how committed are you to investing in yourself? If you don't take the time to care for your own health and wellbeing, you will eventu-ally lose your ability to be of service to anyone else. Don't fall into the trap of thinking that self-sacrifice to the point of exhaustion and poor health is a badge of super-spirituality. Yes, you are called to serve. Yes, you are called to put others interests ahead of your own. But you are also called to care for yourself in a way that will allow you to continue doing those things effectively. Take a look at what Jesus had to say to his apostles when they were in a particularly busy season:

> *The apostles returned to Jesus from their ministry tour and told*
> *him all they had done and taught. Then Jesus said, 'Let's go*
> *off by ourselves to a quiet place and rest awhile.' He said this*
> *because there were so many people coming and going that Jesus*
> *and his apostles didn't even have time to eat.*
> —Mark 6:30-31

If you refuse to take time to care for yourself—to *come apart*, as some other translations put it—you will soon come apart at the seams. Or as I like to say, if you do not come apart, you will come apart. Failing to invest in yourself by eating properly, moving your body, resting well and doing the other things required for health will destroy you and your ability to minister to those around you.

I recently heard a story about a lady who called her church's office and asked to speak to the pastor. The secretary said, "I'm sorry, the pastor is not available. Today is his Sabbath. He'll be in tomorrow." The following Sunday, that lady marched up to the pastor, got right in his face and said, "I really needed to talk to you last week and your secretary said you were taking the day off! Satan doesn't take a day off!" The pastor responded, "You are exactly right. He doesn't. And if I don't take a day off, I'm going to end up just like Satan." The same holds true for you and me. We have to care for ourselves to be able to keep living and loving well.

3. Commit to a healthy lifestyle. In order to choose life, you have to adopt a lifestyle that promotes and sustains life. As we've discussed at length, getting healthy takes long-term thinking. It's not something you can accomplish with fad diets or two-week exercise plans. Instead of giving into the temptation for a quick fix, you must commit to an ongoing healthy lifestyle. The best litmus test for whether the changes you are making can be part of such a lifestyle is to ask yourself, "Is this something I could continue doing for the rest of my life?" If the answer is no, then you aren't developing a lifestyle; you're simply on a crash course.

I once had a woman tell me, "Pastor, I have figured out how to take off the extra pounds. I'm on the soup plan. I eat fresh, healthy soups for all of my meals—and my weight is starting to drop!" After weeks of her talking about the soup plan to others in my church who were trying to get healthy, I had to pull the woman aside and clarify the difference between a diet and lifestyle. I asked her if she was planning to eat soup three times a day for the rest of her life. When she said no, I explained that she was not creating a healthy lifestyle; she had simply gone on a diet. This kind of short-term thinking only leads to short-term results.

Lifestyle vs.	Quick Fix
Long Term	Short Term
Custom Made For You	One Size Fits All
Living Food	Pills, Powders, and Potions
Ongoing Exercise Routine	Short-Term Extreme Work Outs
You Enjoy It	You Endure It

As you consider what you've learned in these pages and begin creating a lifestyle that works specifically for you, make sure to focus on the long-term. With every new decision about your health, be sure to ask yourself, "Is this something I can keep up?" If it's not, re-evaluate your approach.

Your healthy lifestyle won't look exactly like mine or like anyone else's. Yes, there are universal rules about eating, exercise and stress reduction that we all need to work within (as we've discussed), but the day-to-day specifics of what you eat and when, how you get your exercise, and how you make time to rest will be unique to you. Keep those specifics conducive to your long-range goals. Focus on small steps every day and watch your life transform.

4. Decide to maximize your impact. God gave you life so that you could make a difference. Still, as believers, you and I don't always feel at home in this world. We long for the sweetness of heaven. As Paul wrote:

I'm torn between two desires: I long to go and be with Christ, which would be far better for me. But for your sakes, it is better that I continue to live. Knowing this, I am convinced that I will remain alive so I can continue to help all of you grow and experience the joy of your faith.
—Philippians 1:23-25

In this passage, Paul is essentially saying that he is choosing life—not just for his own benefit, but so that he can positively influence those coming behind him. In the same way, you and I must choose life so that we can impact those who have been placed in our paths. People who choose to neglect their health, ending up sick and struggling to get through each day, rarely have much impact on the world. And dead people have even less. By deciding to get healthy, you are taking a major step toward maximizing the difference your life can make now and in generations to come. Consider this passage:

> *Only take heed to yourself, and diligently keep yourself, lest you forget the things your eyes have seen, and lest they depart from your heart all the days of your life. And teach them to your children and your grandchildren.*
> —Deuteronomy 4:9 (NKJV)

Do you have children? Do you have grandchildren? Even if you don't right now, it's likely that one day God will bless you with both. When that day comes, you owe it to them to be healthy and vibrant, ready and able to engage with them well. You owe it to yourself to be able to participate in their lives at full capacity for as long as possible.

When my (Steve's) first granddaughter was born, my motivation for getting healthy increased exponentially. Being able to live life with her, love her and teach her the things of God suddenly meant so much more to me than any greasy cheeseburger or bowl of ice cream ever could. I've come to realize that the things that rob me of my health also rob me of my potential to live and love well—and they are just not worth it. They'll never be worth it again. The short-term pleasure that unhealthy foods and inactivity may give me isn't worth missing out on lasting memories with my family.

Living for Today, Tomorrow and Eternity

One day—on the day you meet the Lord—you will receive a glorified body. As scripture teaches, there will be no more pain and no more suffering (Revelation 21:4). You will be whole and eternally healthy. What a glorious day that will be. But until that day comes, you have a responsibility, a calling even, to take care of the earthly vessel God has given you in a way that shines his excellence; to make it a vessel of honor and strength, capable of accomplishing every task he has called you to. I pray that with God's help you will make the daily choices that will allow that to happen. Choose to live in such away that will allow you to experience the abundance God offers today, to impact the people around you for a better tomorrow, and to alter eternity in a positive way forevermore.

It's time to get healthy, Renegade Pastor. Are you ready? Don't settle for average. Don't let anyone or anything convince you that you are only capable of second best when it comes to your physical wellbeing. God has given you strength; nurture it. He has given you vitality; protect it. He has given you opportunity; stay well so you can fulfill it. Choose to step apart from the crowd and live a better life. Choose to go renegade with every aspect of your health. When you do, God will be able to do more in you and through you than you've ever imagined.

Now all glory to God, who is able, through his mighty power at work within us, to accomplish infinitely more than we might ask or think. Glory to him in the church and in Christ Jesus through all generations forever and ever! Amen.
—Ephesians 3:20-21

Small Steps to Life

- Decide to stop procrastinating. Make it a point to eat something healthy and do some type of exercise today.

- Look back through this book and identify the *Small Steps to Life* that most resonate with you. Write down the ones that you want to begin implementing right away.

- Think about the people who motivate you to live a healthier life. Is it your wife? Your children? Your grandchildren? Put a picture of that person or those people in a place where you'll see it often. Focus on getting healthy so you can spend much more quality time with them in the years to come.

- Spend some time reflecting on all you've learned as you've read these pages. Ask God to direct you and show you his grace as you begin stepping into your new healthy lifestyle.

• • •

A final personal note from Nelson, Steve and Jennifer:
We hope this book will be the beginning of an ongoing conversation. Please visit HealthyRenegade.com to connect with us, receive our free resources or share your story.

How to Set Up Your Losing to Live Group Competition

Can people lose weight without a group competition? Yes, they can, but most people do much better when they are part of a community environment. Getting healthy with a larger group provides support that goes a long way during those initial efforts at weight loss. We all need connection and a place to share our successes and failures. So don't try to lose weight alone and don't ask your church to either — create teams of losers! Here is a simple guide for setting up a *Losing to Live* Weight Loss Competition.

What to Do Before the Competition

Step 1: Know Your Purposes

If you are clear about your purposes and can articulate them to key leaders and to your congregation, you will quickly gain their approval. Christians are the most overweight people group in America, and *Losing to Live* has been designed to confront and help solve this problem. The program will show people in your church how to lose weight and keep it off. The goal is to change lives one pound at a time.

Step 2: Seek Approval from the Leadership of Your Church

- If you are the pastor, inform your key leaders about what you are planning to do and why you are doing it.

- If you are not the pastor, go first to your pastor and share your passion to help church members lose weight. Then let the pastor inform the key leaders.

Step 3: Establish Your Schedule and Location

Any time of year is a good time to start a *Losing to Live* competition because overweight people think about their weight struggle almost every day. The entire competition takes twelve weeks. Participants meet once a week for ninety minutes. During the first thirty minutes, everyone watches a *Bod4God* video and gets an update on the total weight loss results. During the remaining sixty minutes, participants break into teams for discussion. You will need:

- A place that is large enough for all of the participants to meet together and that is equipped to play the *Bod4God* videos.

- Smaller rooms or areas where individual teams can meet.

- A private place to put your scale for weigh-ins.

Step 4: Recruit and Assign Leaders

You'll want to recruit a director, team captains and administrative support to do the weigh-ins and other activities during the sessions. Pray earnestly about who these people should be, as they will be crucial to the success of the program.

Step 5: Organize Your Registration Process

All participants must fill out a *Losing to Live* Registration Form. The form is part of the *Bod4God* Video Series Kit and can be found at Bod4God.org. This form will help you in ordering your participant kits, organizing your teams, and communicating with your participants.

Step 6: Implement Your Promotion Strategy

Your promotion should target your church and your community. A promotional video and other materials are available in the *Bod4God* Video Series Kit, which can be obtained at Bod4God.org.

Step 7: Host an Orientation Meeting

Two to three weeks before the first competition, host an orientation meeting for potential participants. The goal of the meeting is to explain how the competition works and then register participants for the upcoming twelve-week competition. Distribute the *Losing to Live* Fact Sheet and show the Orientation Video presentation by Pastor Steve Reynolds, both of which are part of the *Bod4God* Video Series Kit and can be found at Bod4God.org.

Step 8: Order Your Participant Kits

Each participant should receive an official *Losing to Live* Weight Loss Participant Kit (available at Bod4God.org). The kit contains a copy of the *Bod4God* book by Pastor Steve Reynolds (each participant will need a book to do the Victory Guide exercises that are a crucial element to success in the program), an official *Losing to Live* T-shirt and Refrigerator Magnet.

Step 9: Determine Your Teams

After each participant has been registered, divide the enrollees into teams of six to twelve people. Each team should be balanced out between those who need to lose a lot of weight and those who need to lose less weight. Don't worry if you only have one or two teams the first time. As these first teams have success, others will notice and join the program.

Step 10: Set Up Your Weigh-In Procedure

You will need a good-quality scale and a private place for weigh-ins. Setting up the scale in a classroom is often ideal. To respect everyone's privacy, have participants come in one at a time to weigh in. For the convenience of the participants, the best time to schedule weigh-ins is before and after the meetings. The weight loss competition is based on the percentage of weight lost, not the number of pounds lost. Most groups use a Microsoft Office Excel spreadsheet to do their calculations.

Step 11: Set Up How You Will Communicate with Participants

Get email addresses and phone numbers from all participants. For the best success, the director and the group leader need to be in contact with the participants on a weekly basis. A little encouragement will go a long way toward helping the participants stay on track.

What to Do During the Competition

Step 1: Conduct Weekly Weigh-Ins

Record the participants' weights each week without comment. Whether they have lost or gained, this is their story to tell. Say nothing to the participant or to anyone else.

Step 2: Conduct Weekly Rally Time

At the rally, announce the total weight loss, individual teams' total weight loss, and some of the top individual losers. Show the *Bod4God* video that goes with the weekly chapter in the *Bod4God* book. (The *Bod4God* Video Series Kit is available at Bod4God.org).

Step 3: Conduct Weekly Small Groups

Most participants will connect best with the program within their small group teams. Each team should choose a team name based on a fruit or vegetable as a rallying cry. During each team meeting, the participants should:

- Go over the information in *Bod4God* chapter by chapter.

- Specifically discuss the weekly Victory Guide assignments, including their Small Steps to Life.

- Share ideas on what works and what doesn't work for each person.

- Cheer each other's successes.

- Pray together.

Step 4: Conduct a Victory Celebration

Although the weekly rally time is a kind of celebration, you will also want to have a big, final celebratory event. Note that:

- During this last-week celebration, you will change the order of the meeting by having the small group time first and the rally time second. (The small groups will meet first to go over the material from week twelve.)

- You will announce the overall weight loss for the group and the various teams during the celebration and recognize the individual biggest loser(s).

- Give each participant a certificate of participation (available in the *Bod4God* Video Series Kit).

- You should decide if you would like to give out prizes.

- Any food provided for this event should be healthy.

- If you have individuals who have had unusual success, you may want to call in the media to do a story.

- Rejoice over what God has helped you accomplish together and make sure everyone leaves feeling like a winner.

For more information or to get a complete *Losing to Live* Weight Loss Competition Group Starter Kit, which includes the *Bod4God* book, *Bod4God* Video Series, official *Losing to Live*

T-shirt, and refrigerator magnet, visit Bod4God.org or contact:

Losing to Live
P.O Box 300
Merrifield, VA 22116
703-635-7100 • 866-596-6008

You may also contact Pastor Steve Reynolds about speaking to your church or organization.

Acknowledgements

Nelson Searcy: First and foremost, I would like to thank Jesus Christ for the opportunity to serve his church. I would also like to thank my co-authors on this book. This is my first book with Steve Reynolds. His influence in my life goes well beyond the words on these pages. Thank you, Steve, for your friendship, influence and passion—and especially for your willingness to model the Healthy Renegade Pastor lifestyle.

This is my fourteenth book with Jennifer Dykes Henson. Thank you, Jennifer, for your ongoing commitment to our writing ministry and for your passion for health and wellness; it shines through these pages!

I must also express my appreciation to the staff and members of The Journey Church; the alumni from my coaching networks who shared their testimonies and assisted in the ideas developed in this book; and the entire team at Church Leader Insights, especially Scott Whitaker, Sandra Olivieri and Jimmy Britt.

My passion to live a Healthy Renegade lifestyle is first and foremost about obedience to scripture and my intention to fulfill God's call upon my life. But a close second to that is my desire to honor my marriage to Kelley and to be a healthy parent to my son, Alexander—I love you both! Now, off to my morning run....

Steve Reynolds: I am so thankful to God for using His Word, the greatest health book, to transform me into a healthy renegade pastor. It was an honor to write this book with Nelson Searcy and Jennifer Dykes Henson. Nelson is a much-valued friend and coach. He has literally influenced my life from the top of my head, the way I think, to the bottom of my feet, the shoes I wear. Jennifer's skill in writing and knowledge about health added so much to the quality of this book. I am deeply grateful for Jana Moritz, my writing assistant, who helped me with this book and my two previous books. I am so blessed to have the support of my Capital Baptist Church family and the Losing to Live family. I plan to continue as a healthy renegade pastor, hoping to live a very long time. I want to be on this earth as long as possible with my precious wife and all our precious children and grandchildren!

Jennifer Dykes Henson: Honoring God through health and wellness is a true passion of mine. Having the opportunity to pour all that I've learned and experienced in my own health journey into these pages has been nothing short of a labor of love.

Thank you, Nelson, for once again allowing me to partner with you in creating material that will influence lives in the here and now for the better, and impact the kingdom in unseen ways. Every project we work on together is more exciting than the last!

Thank you, Steve, for all that you do to turn the tide on the health epidemic robbing our churches and their people of the lives they're meant to live. You are a true torchbearer. Your impact in the realm of health and wellness cannot be overstated. It has been a pleasure to work on this book with you.

Thanks also to my husband, Brian, for being a constant source of love and support. To Isabelle and her soon-to-be baby sister, thank you for inspiring your dad and me to live the healthiest lives possible, so that we can enjoy every one of your tomorrows with you.

Finally, thanks to God for giving me the chance to engage in meaningful work that will, hopefully and prayerfully, touch the lives of those who find it in their hands for the better.

Notes

Chapter 1—A Tale of Two Pastors

1. Finkelstein, Eric, et al. "Obesity and Severe Obesity Forecasts Through 2030." *American Journal of Preventive Medicine*. 1 June 2012. Web. 3 Aug. 2014.
2. *Ibid.*
3. Carroll, Jackson, Becky McMillan, and John James, Jr. "Selected Findings From the National Clergy Survey." *Pulpit and Pew*. 1 Feb. 2002. Web. 4 Aug. 2014.
4. Wells, Bob. "Which Way to Clergy Health?" *Pulpit & Pew*. 1 Sept. 2002. Web. 4 Aug. 2014.
5. *Ibid.*
6. Nack, R.A. *Work-in-Text for Earl Nightingale's Lead the Field*. Chicago: Nightingale-Conant, 1974.

Chapter 3—Surrender Your Body to God

1. Warren, Rick, Daniel Amen, and Mark Hyman. *The Daniel Plan: 40 Days to a Healthier Life*. Grand Rapids, Michigan: Zondervan, 2013. p. 20.

Chapter 6—Ten Commandments for Healthy Living

1. "Jesus Walking." Web. 1 Sept. 2014.
   <http://keyboardsforchrist.com/Sandals.html>.

Chapter 7—Exposing the Acceptable Sin

1. Russell, Rex. *What the Bible Says About Healthy Living*. 2nd ed. Ventura, Calif., U.S.A.: Regal, 2006. p. 37.

Chapter 8—How Renegades Eat
1. Rubin, Jordan. *The Maker's Diet*. New York: Penguin Group, 2004. p. 31.
2. Fuhrman, Joel. *Eat to Live: The Amazing Nutrient-Rich Program for Fast and Sustained Weight Loss*. Rev. ed. New York: Little Brown, 2011. p. 82.
3. *Ibid*, p.88.
4. Salmeron, J, et al. *Dietary Fiber, Glycemic Load, and Risk of NIDDM in Men*. U.S. National Library of Medicine, 1 Apr. 1997. Web. 5 Sept. 2014.
5. *2014 National Diabetes Statistics Report*. Centers for Disease Control and Prevention, 24 Oct. 2014. Web. 5 Sept. 2014.
6. Fuhrman, Joel. *Eat to Live: The Amazing Nutrient-Rich Program for Fast and Sustained Weight Loss*. Rev. ed. New York: Little Brown, 2011. p. 50.
7. *Ibid*, p. 114
8. *Ibid*, p. 115.

Chapter 9—Avoid Common Pitfalls
1. Pressfield, Steven. *Do the Work! Overcome Resistance and Get Out of Your Own Way*. Hastings, NY: Do You Zoom, 2011. p. 6, 8-9.

Chapter 10—Drink Up
1. "Why Drinking Water Is Important for Weight Loss." *Calories per Hour*. Web. 6 Sept. 2014.
2. Colbert, Don. *The Seven Pillars of Health: The Natural Way To Better Health for Life*. Lake Mary, FL. Charisma Media, 2007. p. 31.

Chapter 11—Made to Move

1. Kresser, Chris. "How Sitting Too Much Is Making Us Sick and Fat—And What to Do About It." *The Huffington Post.* 18 Mar. 2013. Web. 2 Aug. 2014.
2. "Sedentary Lifestyle Is Dangerous to Your Health: NCHPAD - Building Inclusive Communities." *National Center on Health, Physical Activity and Disability (NCHPAD).* Web. 12 Sept. 2014.
3. Rubin, Jordan. *The Maker's Diet.* New York: Penguin Group, 2004. p.174
4. "Sedentary Lifestyle Statistics." *LifeSpan Blog.* 27 Mar. 2013. Web. 1 Oct. 2014.

Chapter 12—Know Your Numbers

1. Fuhrman, Joel. *Eat to Live: The Amazing Nutrient-Rich Program for Fast and Sustained Weight Loss.* Rev. ed. New York: Little Brown, 2011. p. 31.
2. *Ibid,* p. 30.
3. *Ibid,* p. 31.

Chapter 14—How Renegades Sleep

1. Jones, Maggie. "How Little Sleep Can You Get Away With?" *The New York Times.* 16 Apr. 2011. Web. 5 Oct. 2014.
2. Jones, Jeffrey. "In U.S., 40% Get Less Than Recommended Amount of Sleep." *Gallup.* 19 Dec. 2013. Web. 5 Oct. 2014.
3. Griffin, R. Morgan. "Sleep and Health: 9 Surprising Reasons to Get More Sleep." *WebMD.* Web. 1 Oct. 2014.

Chapter 16—Honor the Sabbath
1. Spurgeon, C.H. *The Preacher's Power and the Conditions of Obtaining It: The Sword and the Trowel.* Liskeard, Cornwall, UK: Diggory Press, 2007.

Chapter 17—From Stress to Rest
1. "Stress Symptoms: Effects of Stress on the Body." *WebMD.* Web. 9 Oct. 2014.

Chapter 18—Maintain Your Emotional Health
1. "Improving Emotional Health: Strategies and Tips for Good Mental Health." *HelpGuide.org.* Web. 12 Oct. 2014.
2. "Mind/Body Connection: How Your Emotions Affect Your Health." *FamilyDoctor.org.* Web. 12 Oct. 2014.
3. Zylstra, Sarah. "1 in 4 Pastors Have Struggled with Mental Illness, Finds LifeWay and Focus on the Family." *Christianity Today.* 22 Sept. 2014. Web. 12 Oct. 2014.

Chapter 19—Forgive Your Enemies
1. Desjardins, Sylvain-Jacques. "Can Blaming Others Make People Sick?" *Concordia University.* 9 Aug. 2011. Web. 20 Oct. 2014.
2. "Research Links Cancer with Repressed, Unresolved Feelings and Emotions." *Examinor.com.* 7 Oct. 2009. Web. 12 Oct. 2014.

Chapter 20—Shrink Your Church
1. Ferraro, Ken. "Study Finds Some Faithful Less Likely to Pass the Plate." *Purdue University*. 24 Aug. 2006. Web. 21 Oct. 2014.
2. Paul, Maria. "Religious Young Adults Become Obese By Middle Age." *Northwestern University*. 23 Mar. 2011. Web. 21 Oct. 2014.

Chapter 21—Lose to Live
1. "YMCA." *Wikipedia*. Wikimedia Foundation, 12 Jan. 2014. Web. 29 Oct. 2014.

How HEALTHY is Your Church?

Learn the Eight Systems of Your Church With Your FREE COPY of Nelson Searcy's *Healthy Systems, Healthy Church* e-book!

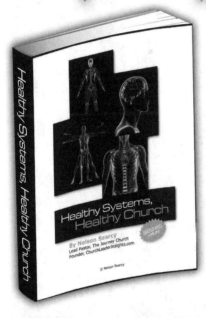

God designed all the parts of the body – both the church body and the physical body – to work together, allowing us to fulfill his purposes and plans on this earth. And both of those respective bodies function best through well-developed systems.

Nelson Searcy's revised *Healthy Systems, Healthy Church* e-book has been updated to include diagnostic questions for you to determine the current health of your church's systems and practical help as you lead your church to greater health and effectiveness.

Download your FREE e-book now ($23.95 value):
www.ChurchLeaderInsights.com/systems

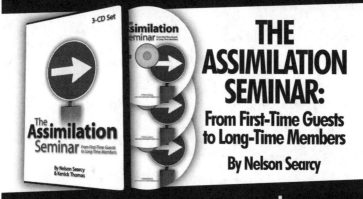

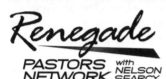
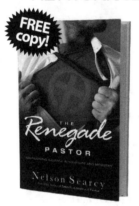

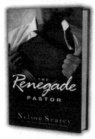
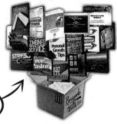